I0073160

QUINTESSENCE OF PHARMACOVIGILANCE

QUINTESSENCE OF PHARMACOVIGILANCE

Prof (Dr.) Tapan Kumar Chatterjee
M. Pharm. (J.U), Ph.D (J.U.), FIC (Cal.).,ARSC(Lond.)

Ex. Research Scientist (UGC),
Department of Pharmceutical Technology,
Jadavpur University, Kolkata.

Director,
Clinical Research Centre (CRC),
Department of Pharmaceutical Technology,
Jadavpur University, Kolkata.

Professor,
Division of Pharmacology,
Department of Pharmaceutical Technology,
Jadavpur University, Kolkata.

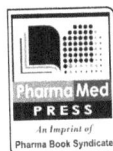

PharmaMed Press
An imprint of Pharma Book Syndicate
A unit of BSP Books Pvt. Ltd.
4-4-309/316, Giriraj Lane,
Sultan Bazar, Hyderabad - 500 095.

Quintessence of Pharmacovigilance *by*
Prof (Dr.) Tapan Kumar Chaterjee

© 2017, *by Publisher*

No part of this book or parts thereof may be reproduced, stored in a retrieval system or transmitted in any language or by any means, electronic, mechanical, photocopying, recording or otherwise without the prior written permission of the publishers.

Published by

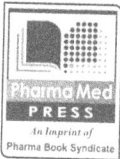

PharmaMed Press

An imprint of Pharma Book Syndicate

A unit of BSP Books Pvt. Ltd.

4-4-309/316, Giriraj Lane, Sultan Bazar, Hyderabad - 500 095.

Phone: 040-23445600/688; Fax: 91+40-23445611

E-mail: info@pharmamedpress.com

ISBN: 978-93-8681-956-7 (HB)

This book is dedicated to my loving daughter

'ANUJA'

PROFESSOR A. N. BASU
EMERITUS PROFESSOR OF PHYSICS
AND
FORMER VICE-CHANCELLOR
JADAVPUR UNIVERSITY

যাদবপুর বিশ্ববিদ্যালয়

*JADAVPUR UNIVERSITY
KOLKATA-700 032, INDIA

DEPARTMENT OF PHYSICS

PRELUDE

I am happy to note that the 1st edition of the book "Quintessence of Pharmacovigilance" is being published and I am sure that this compilation will also serve to satisfy as well as generate further curiosity among all the readers of clinical field.

With the materialization of adverse drug reactions after the treatment of wide spectrum of human disease, a basic understanding of Pharmacovigilance is essential for medical and pharmaceutical student as well as clinicians.

Prof. (Dr.) Tapan Kumar Chatterjee, Professor of Department of Pharmaceutical Technology of Jadavpur University has made a commendable work in bringing out this compilation on *Pharmacovigilance.* In this book, Prof. Chatterjee has included important chapters on prescription errors, adverse drug reactions, drug-drug interactions which highlight the necessity of Pharmacovigilance. He has also included in this book the present Indian and global scenario of Pharmacovigilance. The book will be a useful tool for medical and pharmacy students, medical practitioners, pharmacologists, nurses and toxicologists.

Prof. A. N. Basu
Ex. Vice-Chancellor
Jadavpur University

Kolkata – 700 032

PREFACE

After more than a decade of experience of clinical research activities, publication of significant clinical data on Pharmacovigilance and conducting of courses and seminars on clinical pharmacology I personally felt a need to assimilate my experiences with current emerging trends in Pharmacovigilance in this book. Pharmacovigilance is a rapidly growing area of clinical pharmacy in recent times. During the course of my professional career I felt there was a need for illumination of the subtle relationship between Pharmacovigilance and prescription errors, Adverse Drug Reactions, Drug-Drug interactions in a single publication for the pharmaceutical professionals. This book represents a collection of relevant topics of interest on pharmacovigilance from exhaustive literature searches and personal professional experiences. This book should serve as a useful tool and reference guide in Pharmacovigilance for pharmaceutical professionals.

"**Quintessence of Pharmacovigilance**" is expected to be a reference guide for medical and pharmaceutical students at undergraduate and postgraduate levels. It would also improve awareness about the importance of Pharmacovigilance in clinical practice. The book has five chapters. **Chapter I** deals with Prescription errors which may result in adverse drug reactions. **Chapter II** elaborates all about the Pharmacovigilance of Adverse Drug reactions. **Chapter III** discusses Drug-drug interactions. **Chapter IV** includes Good Pharmacovigilance Practice (GPP) and **Chapter V** looks the current state of Indian and global Pharmacovigilance.

Every effort has been made to maintain the authenticity of the discussed topics and their relevant references in this book for the convenience of the readers. However, any thoughtful additions or improvements to the discussed topics herein, from additional experts, are also welcome to make this publication even more current and valuable for intended health care professionals.

The idea of writing this publication has been largely made possible from the constant inspiration from Prof. A. N. Basu, ex. Vice Chancellor of our University who despite his current busy schedules and other important responsibilities has been gracious enough to write a foreword for this book. I am also indebted for the help and support from additional faculty members of our University whose constant support and encouragements were indispensable for the successful completion of this effort.

A special gratitude goes to Prof. Biswajit Mukherjee, Head of the Department, Dept. of Pharmaceutical Technology, Prof. A. Samanta, Prof. T. K Maity, Prof. B. Sa, Prof. S. Karmakar, Late Prof. T Sen, Dr. P. Halder, Dr. S. Dewenjee, Senior faculty members of the Department of Pharmaceutical Technology, Jadavpur University.

This book is also a result of enormous encouragements and sacrifices made by my family. Support from my wife (Lisa) and daughter (Anuja) has been a determining factor in enabling me to write this book. My late father (who wrote more than 80 informative articles in journals) was also one of my role models for me in providing me the courage to undertake this challenging endeavour.

I also appreciate the sincere and professional support of Ms. Sharmily Chakraborty, M.Pharm (Clinical) for the editorial support for compiling the final edition of this publication.

I am also grateful to my publisher "BSP Books Pvt. Ltd." and to their editorial staff for their co-operation, encouragement and valuable suggestions. I hope this book will be useful for students, researchers and teachers in expanding their horizons in Pharmacovigilance in the modern era.

It would have been impossible to complete this book without the valuable assistance and useful suggestions of Mr. Biswajit Das, Mr. Saumen Karan, Mr. Saswata Banerjee, Mr. Souvik Debnath, Mr. Biplab Chakra, Mr. Debjyoti Naskar, Ms. Soumita Goswami and Mr. Sudipta Biswas in the editing towards the final versions of this book and the added sketches. I sincerely thank them all for their unwavering assistance in this effort.

It is my hope that **"Quintessence of Pharmacovigilance"** would provide as a ready reference guide for this topic for the entire health care community in years to come.

- Author

CONTRIBUTORS

Prof. (Dr.) Abhijit Sen Gupta (B.Pharm., Ph.D)

Prof. Sen Gupta at present is working as Director cum Principal of Guru Nanak Institute of Pharmaceutical Science and Technology since November 2005. After completion of his graduation from the Department of Pharmaceutical Technology, Jadavpur University he joined as Chief Chemist (Manufacturing) in M/s Don Pharmaceuticals (P) Ltd., Harinavi, West Bengal and worked there from December 1979 to June 1981. Prof Sen Gupta worked as Chief Pharmacist of Ben Seena Hosptial, Hail, Kingdom of Saudi Arabia from December 1989 to February 1993 and then from June 1996 to October 1999 (he was granted leave for this period by Fatima College of Pharmacy). After returning from Kingdom of Saudi Arabia, he did his Ph.D. degree from Jadavpur University. He also worked as Principal of Himalayan Pharmacy Institute, Sikkim from June 2000 to July 2004 and Principal of Netaji Subhash Chandra Bose Institute of Pharmacy, Chakdah, Nadia, West Bengal from August 2004 to November 2005. He has published several original research papers in reputed national and international journals.

Aritra Bhattacharyya (M.Sc)

Aritra Bhattacharyya is presently a Ph.D student at Humboldt University zu Berlin, Germany and guest scientist at Charity University, Berlin, Germany (one of Europe's largest Hospital University) where he is working on infectious disease. After completing his bachelors from Presidency College, Kolkata and masters from Calcutta University, he was part time lecturer of biological sciences at the clinical research centre, department of Pharmacy, department of physical education and department of bioscience & Engineering, Jadavpur University, Kolkata.

Dr. Ashoke Kumar Mitra (M.Pharm., PhD)

Dr. Ashoke K. Mitra is a Global Innovative Consultant for Consumer health care product development and strategy for MNCs at Encore-a consortium of open innovation professionals and global experts from across the globe. After completion of his M.Pharm degree from Jadavpur University, he completed his PhD in Pharmacology from Northeast Louisiana State University in the year 1988. Then he joined in post doctoral research as Senior research Associate in Biochemical Pharmacology at University of South Florida from 1988-1992. And subsequently he went onto do further NIH funded research in Drug metabolism and Pharmacokinetics and *In Vitro / In Vivo* Correlations in human drug metabolism as Senior Research Associate in University of Washington from 1992-1994. Thereafter, he joined The Procter and Gamble Company and worked there as a life science professional in various capacities including as an External Relations Manager for three established P&G brands (i.e. Vicks, Therma Care heatwraps, and PUR water filters) for over 3 years. Responsiblities in this role included monitoring external trends affecting these brands and defining appropriate corporate messages in response to external enquiries and managing crisis as and when appropriate, also defined a new process of the understanding consumer behavior towards these brands through the consumer relations organizations (i.e. 1-800 comments lines). He was also selected as Professional and Scientific Relations Manager at P&G Pharmaceuticals for more than 5 years. Managed a US professional relations program for pre-market conditioning for a new Rx product for osteoporosis treatment. Developed new approaches of osteoporotic patient care needs in collaboration with over 200 physicians and allied health care professionals across the US prior to launch. Some of these patient care approaches were adopted by P&G marketing and sales for inclusion in promotional and sales materials

Mr. Biswajit Das (M.Pharm)

Mr. Biswajit Das is a well known teacher as well as researcher in the field of pharmacy. He obtained his bachelor's and master's degrees in pharmacy from Jadavpur University. He has also succeeded in the entrance examination of NIPER. He worked as an Assistant Professor in various pharmacy institutes for almost four years with a good track record. He was selected as a UGC Junior Research Fellow and continued his scientific research at this level for the last four years. He has published in both national and international reputed journals and authored additional books in pharmacy. He is also an established examiner in the field of pharmacy. Novel research work in Drug delivery, Pharmacology and Toxicology are his core areas of research interest. Presently he is Assistant Professor at Adamas University, Barasat, Kolkata.

Mrs. Farhana Rizwan (M.Pharm)

Farhana Rizwan has completed her Master of Pharmacy from University of Science and Technology, Chittagong (USTC), Bangladesh. At present she is doing PhD program in Jadavpur University, Kolkata, India. She is at present working as an Assistant Professor in the Department of

Pharmacy in East West University (EWU), Dhaka, Bangladesh. She is involved in research areas of interest in the public health sector. She is also involved in designing clinical studies. She has multiple published articles in reputed international and national peer-reviewed journals. She has also published three books from different publishing houses from abroad.

Dr. J. Rajan Vedasiromoni (M.Sc., PhD.)

Dr. Rajan Vedasiromoni, an eminent researcher, has worked as Scientist "G" in the field of both core and applied pharmacology. He has done extensive research work as CSIR research fellow and Scientific Assistant in IIEM, Kolkata. Currently he is Placement coordinator and Registrar in National Institute of Pharmaceutical Education and Research, Kolkata. As a member of Indian Pharmacological Society and Association of Physiologists and Pharmacologists of India, he has multiple contributions in the field of applied pharmacology like Clinical Research, Pharmacovigilance etc. He has published several research papers in national and international journals of repute. He has also mentored both undergraduate and postgraduate students in Pharmacology and contributed towards four chapters in multiple books.

Dr. Pinaki Dutta (MBBS, DNB, FRAS Fccs, CCEBDM, CCGDM, ACMDS)

Dr. Pinaki Dutta is a medical graduate from National Medical College, Kolkata. He has completed his DNB in Medicine from Vivekananda Institute of Medical Science, Kolkata. Additional certificate courses in diabetes and thyroid disorders were obtained from Public Health Foundation of India, Govt. of India. He has more than ten years of experience in clinical practice working in Vivekananda Institute of Medical Sciences and AMRI Hospitals, Kolkata. He has worked as guest faculty for Pharmacovigilance and Clinical Research in Jadavpur University. He is also a life member of Royal Asiatic Society. An Academic Registrar, he has managed to teach both medical and pharmaceutical students. He has also worked in the field of clinical research.

Mr. Prasanta Kumar Chakrabarti (Bsc., M.Pharm, MBA, FIC)

Mr. Prasanta Kumar Chakrabarti has worked for thirty years in major pharmaceutical industry including MNC's as Director (Technical) , Vice President and Senior Vice President in Pharmaceutical Technology Management at the corporate level. He has published several research papers in both national and international journals of repute. He has also published several US and Indian patents in product and process related areas. He holds corporate membership with Controlled Release Society Inc, USA, International Society for Pharmaceutical Engineers (ISPE), USA, and the Indian Pharmaceutical Association (IPA) etc. He has undergone training on Senior Management with McKinsey & Co., USA, Indian Institute of Management Ahmedabad and Bangalore. He is presently engaged in academics for undergraduate and postgraduate level in Pharmaceutical Technology at West Bengal University of Technology and Jadavpur University for last six years. Mr Chakrabarti has guided more than 50 nos. of M.Pharm thesis during his bright academic career.

Dr. Saquiba Yesmin (M.Pharm, PhD.)

Dr. Saquiba Yesmin is presently working as an Associate Professor of Department of Pharmacy, Faculty of Biological Sciences, Jahangirnagar University, Dhaka, Bangladesh. She has participated in Ethics Teachers' Training Course organised by UNESCO in 2015 and has also worked as Assistant Coordinator for Training program on Quality Management of Pharmaceutical Companies jointly organised by SEDF and CBDS. She received the National Science and Technology (NST) fellowship in 2014-2015 and won "Faculty Research Initiative Grant" for 2008-2009 at Central Queensland University, Rockhampton, Australia. She has published several original research papers in reputed national and international journals. She has also presented several papers in seminar held in Australia, Japan and other countries.

Ms. Sharmily Chakraborty (M.Pharm in Clinical Pharmacy-University Gold Medalist)

Ms. Sharmily Chakraborty is a researcher in the field of Pharmacy and is a gold medalist for M.Pharm (Clinical Pharmacy). At present she in the PhD program in the Department of Pharmacy in Jadavpur University. She has received the DST (West Bengal) Junior Research Fellowship for her PhD research. She acquired valuable Clinical Research experience during her M.Pharm research. She has published her research work both in national and international peer-reviewed journals of repute. She has years of experience in working as clinical pharmacist in different reputed hospitals of Kolkata. She also works as a coordinator in the different certificate courses of Clinical Research Centre, Jadavpur University.

CONTENTS

INTRODUCTION

The World Health Organization (2002) has defined Pharmacovigilance (PV or PhV), as the pharmacological science relating to the collection, detection, assessment, monitoring and prevention of adverse effects with pharmaceutical products. The etymological roots of the word "Pharmacovigilance" are *pharmacon* (Greek word) which means drug and *vigilare* (Latin word) which means to take care. Pharmacovigilance is mainly concerned with Adverse Drug Reactions (ADRs). Adverse Drug Reaction is defined as any response to a drug that is considered noxious and/or unintended. The World Health Organization has established the importance of Pharmacovigilance through its International Drug Monitoring program in response to the thalidomide disaster in 1961. As of 2010, 134 countries have become part of WHO Pharmacovigilance Program. Medication errors such as overdose, misuse and abuse of a drug as well as drug revelation during pregnancy and breastfeeding, are also of attention, even without an adverse event, because they may outcome in an adverse drug reaction. The objective of Pharmacovigilance program is to:

- Progress patient safety in connection with the use of both medicines and medical devices.
- Appraise the effects and risk of medicines.
- Persuade the safe and rational use of medicines.
- Encourage understanding, education and training in Pharmacovigilance programs.

Several factors that contribute to the occurrence of adverse drug reactions followed by Pharmacovigilance include medication errors, drug-drug interactions, drug-food interactions, herb-drug interaction adulterated medicines etc. Lack of accuracy in writing a prescription can develop irrational prescriptions which confuse both patients and other healthcare professionals and leading to a rise towards the inappropriate use of pharmaceuticals. Pharmacovigilance also monitors the inappropriate use of pharmaceuticals without lack of credible scientific evidence. Pharmacovigilance also identifies hazards and complications associated with the use of pharmaceuticals and tries to minimize the risk(s) associated for patients.

A full-bodied Pharmacovigilance program is dependent on information received from patients and healthcare providers via pharmacovigilance agreements (PVAs), as well as other sources such as the medical literature. In fact, prior to commercialization of a pharmaceutical product in most countries, adverse event data received by the license holder (usually a pharmaceutical company) must be submitted to the local drug regulatory authority. Pharmacovigilance efforts usually refer to resources from drug regulatory authorities and pharmaceutical companies. Adverse event (AE) reporting involves the receipt, triage, data entering, assessment, distribution, reporting (if appropriate), and archiving of AE data and appropriate documentations. The incident reports on adverse drug reactions come from spontaneous reports from healthcare professionals or patients (or other intermediaries); solicited reports from patient support programs; reports from clinical or post-marketing studies; reports from literature sources; reports from the media (including social media and websites); and reports that are reported to drug regulatory authorities themselves.

CHAPTER 1

PRESCRIPTION ERROR

Introduction

The art of writing a prescription is an essential skill required by doctors. Medications in prescriptions must be prescribed in such a way where the therapeutic benefits and the risk of harm are properly balanced. The clinical knowledge about drugs and proper process of prescription writing must be improvised at each and every time of writing a prescription. Faults in writing a prescription results in prescribing errors. Prescribing of medications is one of the most important parts of treatment and errors in any segment of prescribing process can significantly affect morbidity and mortality of patients. Although prescribing errors are not always fatal, they can lead to the development of serious adverse events which delays recovery of patients. Before going into the details, different terms like "Prescription", "Prescribing", "Prescription Errors", "Adverse drug events" must be properly distinguished.

*A **prescription** (℞) is a health-care program implemented by a physician or other qualified practitioner in the form of instructions that govern the plan of care for an individual patient*[1].

***Prescribing** is the process of deciding what to prescribe and naming it and the act of writing a prescription*[2].

*A definition states that 'a clinically meaningful **prescribing error** occurs when as a result of a prescribing decision or prescription writing process there is an unintentional significant reduction in the probability of treatment being timely and effective or increase in the risk of harm when compared with generally accepted practice'*[3]

An adverse drug event is an injury from a drug related intervention[4][5].

With rapid development of new drug molecules the prevalence of prescribing errors is increasing enormously. Of all types of medication errors, prescribing error is the most serious. Once an error has been made, unless detected, it will be systematically applied and can result in significant harm or death[6]. Inappropriate Prescribing is particularly an important type of medication error. Prescribing errors occur

3

simultaneously both in hospitals and in general practice. A recent review of the literature concerning prescriptions made by junior doctors in hospitals found the range of reported error rates to be 2-514 per 1000 items prescribed and 4.2-82% of patients or charts reviewed [7] . In United Kingdom hospitals, prescribers make errors in 1.5% of prescriptions[8]; and in primary care errors occur in upto 11% of prescriptions.

Types of Prescription Errors

Prescription errors are generally two types. Mistakes in writing a prescription and ignoring several factors (drug-drug interactions, potentially dangerous adverse drug reactions, contraindications), while using a drug both causes prescription errors.

- **Errors in prescription writing:** The act of writing a prescription is not always as careful as it should be. As prescriptions are considered a permanent and unambiguous record of patient's treatment, it should be written properly and clearly. Errors frequently occur while writing dose, route, quantity, frequency and name of drugs.

  Errors in naming of drugs: Various instances show errors in prescribing due to confusion of drug names. As a drug can be available in various trade names, use of brand names instead of approved generic names during prescribing can create confusion and contribute to errors.

  Errors in dose: Writing a dose of a drug without mentioning its unit (for example- 5 instead of 5 mg or 5 gm or 5 ml) is an error. Drugs that are prescribed in very low or high doses suffer this problem. For example levothyroxine, given as 25 µg or 0.25 mg and piperacillin + Tazobactum as 4.5 gm). For this type of medicine if the dose is not properly written life threatening adverse reactions can occur. Lack of usage of exact strength of dose of a tablet / capsule can also confuse the patient and produce unintentional errors.

  Errors in frequency and route: Frequency and route of administration of drugs are occasionally found omitted in prescription.

  Errors in quantity: Errors of quantity are not very common. Forgetting to state the quantity of dosage form or providing wrong number of medicines often occur.

- **Errors in use of drugs:** Every drug has its own standard dose, route and frequency in specific indications along with contraindications and drug-drug interactions. Any incompliance with standard regimen while using a drug can cause error in drug use. Miscalculation of dosage frequently occur for elderly and young patient. Though many drug-drug interactions are found in literature, the importance of them in causing life threatening reaction is sometimes doubtful. Ignoring a potentially harmful interaction can generate errors. Use of a drug without considering the contraindication can cause exacerbation of existing disease.

Why Prescription Errors do Occur?

Prescription errors are typical events that derive from slips, lapses, mistakes[9]. Several other factors contribute to prescription errors. The main focus of discussing the reasons behind occurrence of prescription errors should be on the prevention of adverse drug events.

➢ **Inadequate drug knowledge:** Lack of clinical knowledge about drugs, their indications, contraindications, appropriate dose, different dosage forms, routes, interactions with other drugs can give rise to errors which results in ineffective therapy or in adverse drug reactions.

- *Drug-drug interactions:* Insufficient knowledge or competence and incomplete information about drugs initiate drug-drug interactions to happen. These can have serious consequences. Polypharmacy or the use of five or more medications in single prescription can induce dug-drug interactions.There are many medications which should be used cautiously with each other. Some of them are given below.

TABLE 1.1

Some potential drug-drug interactions

First Drug	Second Drug	Possible result of Interaction
Amiodarone	Beta-Blockers (Propanolol, Metoprolol)	Bradycardia, Ventricular fibrillation and asystole on abdominal application
	Calcium channel Blockers	Sinus arrest and aerious hypotension occurs

TABLE 1.1 Contd...

First Drug	Second Drug	Possible result of Interaction
Disopyramide	Rifampicin	May cause marked reduction in serum levels on concurrent use.
Aminoglycoside antibiotics (Amikacin)	Cephalosporins (Cefuroxime, cefepime, cefoperazone)	Nephrotoxic effects can be increased by concurrent use.
Isoniazide	Antacids	Absorption of isoniazid may be reduced by concurrent use.
Cefuroxime	Pantoprazole	Absorbtion of cefuroxime is delayed.

Often simultaneous use of prescription drugs and other self-prescribed medicines can cause drug-drug interactions.

Drug-drug interactions can be reduced by updating knowledge about drugs and patient's records.

- **Dosing errors:** Proper dosing is of particular importance in special population of patients like elderly and children. Both in case of elderly and children drugs are dosed based on body surface area, age etc. In case of children, several guidelines are available which states the dose of drug/kg/day. Use of adult dose in children derives potentially harmful adverse drug events. For example-the pediatric dose of amoxicillin is 50 mg/kg/day which can be divided to 6 hours or 8 hours. Care in prescribing drugs for older patients must be taken by doctors. Dosing error occur in elderly patients at the initiation of therapy. For example, an initial dose of hydrochlorothiazide at 6.25 mg/day is effective in elderly but they are often treated with 25 or 50 mg/day which leads to development of side effects like orthostatic hypotension[10][11].

Errors in dosing occur frequently for patients with impaired renal functions and in hepatic failure patients. Drugs whose active forms are renaly cleared, doses of those drugs need to be altered. Renal impairment modifies the effects of many drugs mainly by increasing their effects in the body. Dosing in renal failure patients is done by calculating the glomerular filtration rate / Creatinine Clearance (Creatinine Clearance is calculated by using Cockcroft-gault reaction). Miscalculations of dose in such patients cause accumulation of drugs in the body leading to potential toxicity followed by adverse drug reactions. Hence prescribing of dose in this type of patients need to be proper to prevent harm.

Dose calculation for patients with hepatic failure is more difficult than for patients with impaired renal function. As metabolism of drugs is mainly done by liver, modification of dosing of those drugs need to be remembered. No such formula is available for calculating hepatic dose of drugs. But careful prescribing should be done in patients with liver dysfunction to avoid errors.

- *Errors in indications and contraindications:* During prescribing correct indication of a drug and the particular medical condition in which the drug cannot be prescribed must be known by the prescriber. Prescriber who do not have clear idea about indications and contraindications can cause misuse of drugs.

  Misuse defines the use of drugs that results in unnecessary complications[11][12].

  For example: Aspirin, a popular non-steroidal anti-inflammatory drug and also an anti-platelet drug is Contraindicated in patients with peptic ulcer and also in pediatric population due to risk of development of Reye's syndrome. Caution is needed for prescribing of aspirin in such type of patients.

- *Errors due to use of 'Banned' dugs:* Numerous drugs that cause life threatening phenomenon on prolong use are banned for use either in whole population or in special population. List of banned drugs vary from country to country. In some countries banned drugs are available in the market for sale. Lack of updated knowledge about such kind of drugs may cause illegal use of the drugs by prescriber leading to errors.

➢ **Insufficient patient's information:** Inadequate information related to patients can results in errors leading to adverse drug reactions. Poor maintenance of patient's record containing incomplete or wrong history of allergy and medications work as good source of errors.

- *Undocumented allergy:* Mentioning the allergy profile (either drug or food allergy) of a patient in prescription chart helps to prevent prescribing errors. Previously developed allergy of a patient on application of a drug need to be documented on the drug chart of that particular patient. If drug allergy remains undocumented, the drug can be repeated by prescriber and can become error. It was found in a study that about 12.1% of prescribing errors occur due to inadequate patient history of allergy to the same medication class prescribed repeatedly by prescriber[13]. Antibiotics like Penicillin, Azithromycin, Amoxicillin, Psychotropic drugs, NSAIDs are common allergenic drugs. Allergic skin tests are frequently performed before administration of drugs but this is only practiced for antibiotics than other classes of drugs. Known allergic condition of a patient limits the option for treatment. Allergy history requires confirmation before prescribing procedure. If the patient is not in condition to inform it can be asked to the member authorized by the patient. The original circumstances and the complete event of adverse drug reaction that occurred after application of medication also need to be confirmed because the information of allergy may necessitate further investigation.

- *Unreviewed medication history:* Taking care of the medication history is important to avoid prescription errors. Both for inpatients or hospitalized patients and outpatient's previous drug history is required for further treatment. Drug history or regularly used home medicine has its importance particularly in elderly patients with several co-morbid conditions. Numerous common co-morbidities like hypertension, diabetes, Benign hypertrophy of prostate in males, gout or arthritis and any previous medical intervention or surgery are associated with the use of various drugs. Both the knowledge about patient's home medicine and proper documentation of them is required to prevent errors like occurrence of adverse drug reactions or drug-drug interactions. Apart from allopathic medicines other forms of medicines used by the patient needs inclusion.

Sometimes, discrepancies are found between the drugs that are documented in medication history review chart and drugs that are originally taken by the patients. Such type of incomplete medication history also causes potential errors. Certain drugs like cardiovascular drugs require continuation even with the newly prescribed drugs. Improper medication history can cause discontinuation of them leading to worsening of existing medical condition of patient. The patient himself or any authorized relative of patient can be asked about the home medicine of patient. They can also be called to bring the medications during visit to hospital or clinics. Outpatient medical records can be a good source of patient's drug history though it is not always reliable. Maintenance of an updated list of drugs can be sometimes helpful. Medical reconciliation is a relatively new, time saving and trustful procedure to gather information about drug history followed by prevention of prescription errors.

> **Miscommunication or communication error:** Errors are frequently made by medical professionals (not only doctors but also nurses, pharmacists and other medical staff) because they fail to communicate properly. Illegible handwriting, verbal orders or communication, unnecessary use of unapproved abbreviations, symbols, punctuations, drug names pave the way of producing errors.

Illegible handwriting of the prescriber or of the person who is responsible updating the medication chart day to day can have serious effects on producing errors. In a multidisciplinary care system, the busy schedule and the workload due to multiple number of patients forces a doctor to become negligent about writing a prescription. Unclear handwriting in a prescription is often misread by pharmacists and nurses. On other hand, instructions to patients that are little understood require further confirmation by the prescriber. All these type of accidents due to sloppy handwriting either delays the process of treatment or insists dispensing error or administration error to happen.

Ambiguous and incomplete prescription is another common reason of prescription error. Incomplete prescriptions may cause ambiguity which increases the chances of errors. Errors occur when ambiguous instructions provide information that is different from what the prescriber intended. Apart from causing prescribing errors inadequate information contained in prescription can also cause dispensing error as the pharmacist donot get complete information from the prescriber.

In case of medical emergencies, verbal orders are often taken. When instructions about medicines are given through telephone or any other form of communicator, the person receiving the information either a pharmacist, a nurse or a doctor, even a patient himself donot clearly understand. Secondly even if it is appropriately received by the listener errors can occur during transcribing the information. Misinterpretation of the verbal orders produces errors. There is several sound alike drugs which belong to completely different classes. For example - Clonidine, a sympatholytic drug used to treat hypertension can be misinterpreted as klonopine (also known as clonazepam) which is a psychotropic drug. Another example is Amiodarone, a potassium sparing diuretic is often confused with Amrinone. Even brand names of medicines are so confusing and similar that they are difficult to understand through verbal communication. The person taking verbal orders should spell the order properly while reading it back to the person giving orders.

➤ **Use of abbreviations:** Misinterpretation of abbreviations used by prescriber generate a cascade of errors that can lead to an adverse drug reactions. There are several unapproved abbreviations, symbols and punctuations that get confused with the original ones. Nurses and pharmacists fail to understand such unacceptable abbreviations and commence errors. Table 1.2 and 1.3 contains list of such abbreviations, symbols and punctuations that cause errors.

TABLE 1.2

List of drug name abbreviations causing errors

Abbreviations	Actual Meaning	Misinterpretation
AZT	Zidovudine	Azathioprine or Aztreonam
MTX	Methotrexate	Mitoxantrone
PCA	Procainamide	Patient Control Anaesthesia
HCT	Hydrocortisone	Hydrochlorthiazide
MSO_4	Morphine Sulfate	Magnesium Sulfate
TAC	Triamcinolone	Tetracaine,Cocaine
CPZ	Compazine	Chlorpromazine
HCL	Hydrochloride/ Hydrochloric Acid	Misinterpreted as potassium chloride ('H' is missed as 'k')

The above list is adapted from **"List of Error prone Abbreviations, symbols and punctuations"** of Institute for safe medication practices, 2003.

TABLE 1.3

List of symbols and punctuations causing errors

Abbreviations	Actual Meaning	Misinterpretation
µg	Microgram	Miligram/mg
IJ	Injection	"TV" or Intrajugular

TABLE 1.3 *Contd...*

Abbreviations	Actual Meaning	Misinterpretation
IN	Intranasal	"IM" or "IV"
qhs	Nightly at bedtime	'qhr' or every hour
UD	As directed (ut dictum)	Unit dose
Q1d	Daily	q.i.d/ four times a day
BT	Bedtime	BID/ Twice daily
AD/AS	Right ear/Left ear	OD/OS (right eye/left eye)
Zero After decimal point (eg: 5.0 mg)	5 mg	50 mg as decimal point is not seen
< or >	Greater than and Less than	Often mistaken as opposite of intended
×3 d	For 3 days	3 doses

The above list is adapted from **"List of Error prone Abbreviations, symbols and punctuations"** of Institute for safe medication practices, 2003.

PROPOSED FORMAT OF DOCUMENTING PRESCRIPTION ERROR

PRESCRIPTION ERROR REPORTING FORM

TYPES OF PRESCRIPTION ERROR

- **Patient's name missing**   YES ☐   NO ☐
- **Home Medication chart (incomplete or absent)**   YES ☐   NO ☐
- **Dosage Form Missing**   YES ☐   NO ☐
- **Rote of Administration Missing**   YES ☐   NO ☐
- **Use of unapproved Abbreviations or symbols**   YES ☐   NO ☐
- **Omission of dose, route, frequency or dosage unit** YES ☐   NO ☐
- **Missing information about diluent to be used**   YES ☐   NO ☐
- **Missing information about strength of dose**   YES ☐   NO ☐
- **Any unreadable/ incomplete description (Related to**
- **dose, route, frequency, duration, dilution**
- **of current medicine)**   YES ☐   NO ☐
- **Errors of formulation**   YES ☐   NO ☐
- **Others**   YES ☐   NO ☐

WHO INITIALLY DISCOVERED THE ERROR?
(more than one can be selected)

Physician ☐   Nurse ☐   Pharmacist ☐

Family members of patient ☐   Unable to determine ☐   other ☐

OUTCOME OF THE ERROR

DESCRIPTION OF THE ERROR (Who, when, what and how)
....
....
....
....
....
....

DID THE ERROR CAUSE HARM TO PATIENT?

YES ☐ (If yes them mention the type of harm)   NO ☐

....
Signature of Prescriber   **Signature of Clinical Pharmacist**

Systems Implemented to avoid Prescription Error

> **Computerized entry of physician's medication order:** In the past the handwritten and verbally communicated orders have led to produce errors and injuries to patient. Electronic prescription or CPOE is relatively new implementation to avoid this type of errors.

"Computerized provider order entry (CPOE) refers to any system in which clinicians directly enter medication orders (and, increasingly tests and procedures) into a computer system, which then transmits the order directly to the pharmacy"[14].

Recommendations to prevent prescribing errors have been developed by a number of organizations [15]. To reduce the complexity in writing a prescription automated prescribing process has been included in various recommendations. Computerized entry of physician's order is an effective tool to reduce errors. Every decision regarding prescribing process like drug selection, checking of drug-drug interactions, and calculation of dose can be supported by clinical decision support system to help the prescriber.Compared to paper based prescribing, electronic prescribing can enhance patient's safety and medication compliance by improving accuracy and reduce costs of patients by averted adverse drug events[16]. This system is very fruitful as it reduces time in completion of medical orders. Errors related to handwriting and transcribing can also be reduced by this process. Electronic prescribing also reduces the need of verbal communications and also the time spent on this type communication through phone calls between the prescriber and any other medical staff like nurse, pharmacist, other physician and subsequently the errors produced from oral communications. Even if a single medication chart is aided by an electronic prescribing system it helps to develop an immediate feedback control between prescriber and other medical staff helps through collaboration[17]. The only risk behind using CPOE is that it can introduce new type of errors. Inexperience prescriber can cause slower entry of medications and in emergency condition computerized entry can be slower than person to person communication. Proper training and practical skill is needed to avoid the risk related to CPOE.

> **Medical reconciliation:** Medical reconciliation is relatively new term. It is very helpful in preventing adverse drug reactions and drug-drug interactions that arise from improper history taking by prescriber.

According to the joint commission *"Medical reconciliation is the process of comparing a patient's medication orders to all of the medications that the patient has been taken"*[18].

It is done by preparing two lists and comparing them. One list contains the current medications of the patient and the other list contains the medications to be prescribed for the patient. When a patient is admitted to a hospital with several comorbidities he is already prescribed with several medications. A new health related problem forces him to take other medications prescribed by the prescriber in hospital. When the patient gets discharged from the hospital prescribers often forget to allow them to continue the required home medicines. Medical reconciliation fill the gap between the home medications and patient's current medications in hospital. A home care department of one hospital found that about in their hospital about 77% patients were discharged with inadequate medical instructions[19]. Medical reconciliation is repeatedly performed and updated during admission, transfer, any surgical procedure and even at the time of discharge of patient. In case of patients who do not require hospital stay or patients who only comes to visit doctors in clinics due to relatively minor health problem, medical reconciliation is effective to prevent any unwanted adverse drug reaction and drug-drug interaction. It is very healthy process which includes the physician, nurse, pharmacist, family members of patient and even the patient himself. Errors of mission, errors of drug dosing, therapeutic duplication can be prevented by medical reconciliation. Not only prescription errors, medical reconciliation can prevent the subsequent administration and dispensing errors also. An accurate and complete medical reconciliation require proper communication between the patient and prescriber, proper and updated knowledge about medicine and also sufficient time. Though the process of medical reconciliation is not as straight forward as it sounds, it can be taken as a challenge towards reducing medical errors.

> **Error reporting system:** Monitoring and reporting of errors are final steps of reducing the rate of prescribing errors. In order to reduce incident of adverse drug reactions and drug interactions resulting from prescription errors identification of errors is needed first. Detection is very crucial step in error reporting. After proper identification it should be informed. Due to heavy workload errors are often overlooked by doctors and nurses. Even when they are checked by one of the medical staffs' information do not reach to the prescriber due to communication failure. A study has showed that spontaneous reporting is atleast 10 times less effective in detecting errors and adverse drug reactions than active, system oriented error-reporting process[20]. A clinical pharmacist is an authorized person who can be responsible for reviewing and reporting of errors. He is also responsible for informing the prescriber about error and making them aware. Error reporting is voluntary and confidential[17]. Special computerized monitoring and error reporting system can be implemented.

Audit is another important tool for reducing errors. It is official inspection. Audit is relatively bigger concept and usually done by experts. After several months of monitoring and error reporting audit should be done to check if the monitoring and reporting process was correct or not. Audit also helps to know that if the reporting system has improved the quality of prescribing or not. The reduction rate of prescribing errors can also be detected through audit. Prescription audit helps to understand the drug utilization pattern in a hospital.

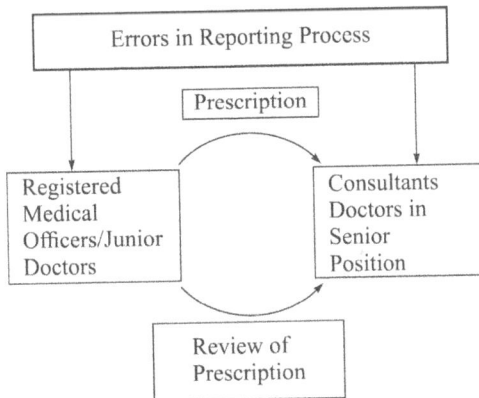

Fig. 1.1 Flow chart showing interventions required to reduce adverse drug reactions.

> **Training, education and organizational intervention:** Prescribing performance can only be improved by proper training and education of doctors prescribing them and also other ancillary medical staffs involved. The complex skill of prescribing requires complete knowledge of the prescriber about medicines and its pharmacology. The improvisational attitude of prescriber towards writing a good prescription is also aided by medical education and training. Education can be done through arrangement of classes on relevant topics. Senior doctors should be involved in teaching. Ancillary medical staff can be trained by junior doctors also. A proper rule of writing a prescription can be maintained which will be followed by every prescriber. All medical staff who deals with prescriptions should be made aware about the policies and guidelines related to medicine. The process of reviewing a prescription is also a concern for good prescribing process and persons responsible for reviewing should also be sufficiently educated. Polypharmacy requires special attention [17]. Different e-learning sources should also be available for the doctors and other staff so that they can improve their professional knowledge about drugs.

Conclusion

Errors in prescription writing and faults in choosing drugs for prescription are preventable most of the times. Proper strategies made regarding the education, monitoring and reporting of errors can reduce errors most of the times. Errors in prescription donot injure the patient all the time. Monitoring of adverse drug reactions concurrently with prescription review also help to prevent further error.

Case Study-1

A prospective observational study was performed by a student on incidence of medication errors in critical care unit in a tertiary care hospital.

He found that drug history error occurred in 10.71% of patients which could lead to prescribing errors. He found that among 196 errors, 21 cases were related to drug history error. He found out of 21 errors 8 (39.09%) were dosing errors. 10 (47.61%) errors were related to frequency and both dosing errors and frequency errors occurred in 3 cases (14.28%)

TABLE 1.4

Table showing errors related to patient's drug history

Frequency errors	47.61%
Dose errors	38.09%
Both	14.28%

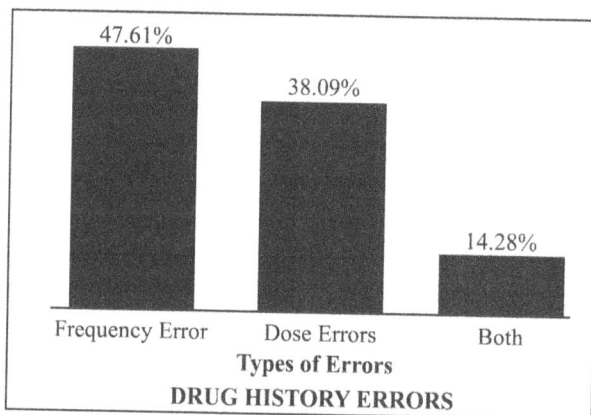

Fig. 1.2 Graph showing errors related to patient's drug history.

It was observed for different types of prescription errors. Among all the errors prescription errors were 20.91%. It was found medication errors happened in 12 cases (29.26%), Frequency errors in 14 cases (34.14%). Route was not mentioned in 13 (31.7%) cases and other types of errors were 4.87 % (2 cases)

TABLE 1.5

Table showing different types of prescription errors

Medication errors	Frequency error	Route not mentioned	Others
12 (29.26%)	14 (34.14%)	13 (31.7%)	2 (4.87%)

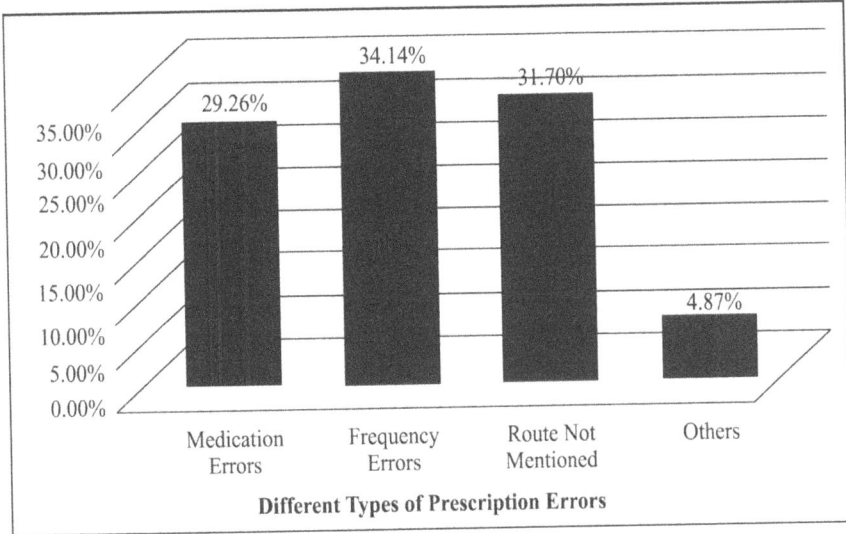

Fig. 1.3 Graph showing different types of prescription errors.

Case Study-2

Another study was also performed in the same hospital. It was prospective observational study on incidence of medication errors in general and surgical ward. Among all patients drug history was not taken in 40 patients (12.38%). Errors were found in medication history chart. 24 patients (14.54%) had drug error, 61 patients (36.97%) had dose error, 15 patients had timing error (9.09%) and 45 patients had combined errors (27.27%). 20 patients (12.12%) had other types of errors (errors in route of administration and duration error).

TABLE 1.6

Table showing errors related to patient's drug history

Drug	Dose	Timing	Combined	Other
24 (14.54%)	61 (36.97%)	15 (9.09%)	45 (27.27%).	20 (12.12%)

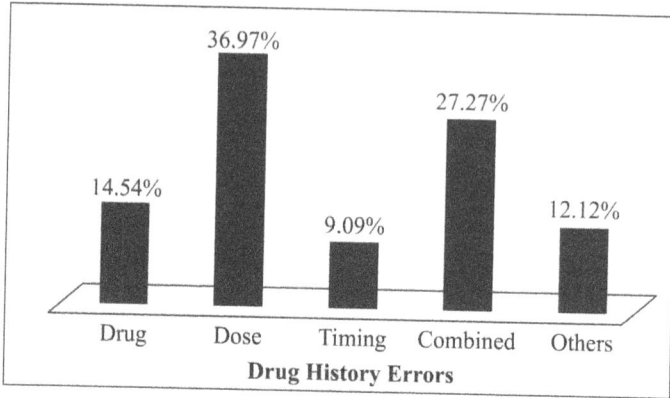

Fig. 1.4 Graph showing errors related to patient's drug history.

In daily prescription chart errors were found. He observed that in medicine card 32 patients (37.20%) medication error, 19 patients (22.09%%) had dosage errors, 22 patients (25.58%) had combined error and 13 patients had other types of errors.(15.11%).

TABLE 1.7

Table showing different types of prescription errors

Medication errors	Dosage errors	Combined errors	Others
32 (37.20%)	19 (22.09%)	22 (25.58%)	13 (15.11%)

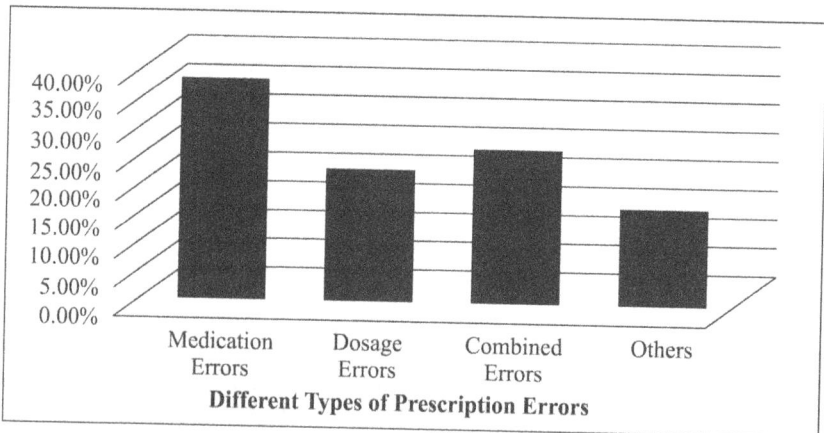

Fig. 1.5 Graph showing different types of prescription errors.

References

1. Agency for Healthcare Research & Quality 2003.

2. Americam Medical Association. (2011). A clinical guide to electronic prescribing. Retrieved December 17, 2011.

3. American society of Hospital Pharmacists. Suggested definitions and relationships among medication misadventures, medication errors, adverse drug events and adverse drug reactions. *Am J Health Syst Pharm*. 1998: 55: 165-66.

4. Beers MH, Berkow R.eds. *The Merck Manual of Geriatrics*.3rd Ed. Whitehouse Station. NJ: Merck Research Laboratories: 2003.

5. Belknap SM, Moore H, Lanzotti SA, Yarnold PR *et al* (September 2008). "Application of software design principles and debugging methods to an analgesia prescription reduces risk of severe injury from medical use of opioids". Clinical Pharmacology & Therapeutics 84.

6. Dean B, Barber N, Schachter M. What is a prescribing error? Qual Health Care 2000; 9: 232-7.

7. Dean B, Schachter M, Vincent C, et al. Prescribing errors in hospital inpatients: their incidence and clinical significance. Qual Saf Health Care2002; 11: 340-4.

8. Flynn EA, Barker KN, Pepper GA, et al. Comparison of methods for detecting medication errors in 36 hospitals and skilled-nursing facilities. *Am J Health Syst Pharm*. 2002: 59: 436-446.

9. Giampaolo P. Velo & Pietro Minuz. Medication Errors: prescribing failts and prescription errors. *Br J Clin Pharmacol*.: 67: 6: 624-628.

10. J D Rozich, M.D, Ph. D. MBA, medication Safety: one organization's approach to the challenge" *Journal of Clinical Outcomes Management,* October 2001, Vol. 8, No. 10, Pages 27-34.

11. Jeffrey K Aronson, Medication errors: definitions and classification. Br J Clin Pharmacol. 2009 Jun; 67(6): 599-604.

12. Jha AK, Kuperman GJ, TEich JM, Leape L, Shea B, Rittenberg E, Burdick E et. al. Identifying adverse drug events: development of a computer based monitor and comparison with chart review and stimulated voluntary report. *J Am Med Inform Assoc*.1998; 5: 305-14.

13. Lesar TS, Bricel and L, Stein d. Factors related to errors in medication prescribing. *JAMA*2003: 289: 1107-1116.

14. Manasse HR Jr. Not too perfect: hard lessons and small victories in patient safety. *Am J Health Syst Pharm*. 2003: 60: 780-787.

15. Micromedex Thomson. MICROMEDEX. All rights reserved. MICRO-MEDEX Healthcare Series. Vol.118 Expired December 2003.

16. N Barber, M Rawlins, B Dean Franklin. Reducing prescribing error: competence, control, and Culture.www.qshc.com

17. Rochon RA, Gurwitz JH. Optimising drug treatment for elderly patient, the prescribing cascade. *BMJ.* 1997: 315: 1096-97

18. Ross S, Bond C, Rothnie H, Thomas S, Macleod MJ. What is the scale of prescribing errors committed by junior doctors? A systematic review. Br J Clin Pharmacol. 2009; 67: 629-40.

19. The Joint Comission. Issue 35: Using medical reconciliation to prevent errors. January 25, 2006.

CHAPTER 2

DRUG INTERACTIONS

PART - A

MODERN DRUG INTERACTION

Introduction

With the increase in number of drugs used for the treatment of an individual the drug therapy has become complicated. One of the main drug-related problems that arise is due to drug interaction where a predictable effect of a drug diminishes. Drug interaction is therefore a condition in which the effects of one drug are altered by prior or concurrent administration of another drug, food or occurrence of any disease state. More conceptually the drug interaction extends to different situations where the drug activity gets influenced by

1. Food or certain dietary items (i.e., drug-food interactions) or
2. Environmental chemicals or smoking
3. Alteration of diagnostic laboratory test results (i.e., drug-laboratory test interactions) or
4. Certain disease states (i.e., drug-disease interactions).

With the increase in drug interaction the subject is been highly focused. In order to deal with the incidence of drug interaction, information is gathered and public awareness is created by publications of articles related to the topic. This drug interaction can either elevate or reduce the response of one or more of the agents used leading to either serious adverse effect or loss of efficacy respectively. Example is the enhanced effect of agents like digoxin and warfarin leading to adverse effects. Even though relevant data is available for different concurrent drug administration, drug interaction occurs. With the increase in number of drugs in a therapeutic regimen of a patient the risk of drug interaction also increases.

Drug Interactions

The drug interaction is an observable fact, which occurs when the effects of one drug are changed by the existence of other drug, food and drink or by some environmental chemical substances. The drug interaction may induce either beneficial or harmful effects. However, adverse or harmful effects are predominated. The mechanism of both types of interactions (beneficial and harmful) is very similar. Here in this chapter we have discussed only the adverse interactions. Drugs can interact with each other at any point from their being mixed during pharmaceutical formulation upto their final stage of excretion from the body. The more the number of drugs a patient takes, the greater will be the chances of adverse reactions. Many drugs which are known to interact in some patients simply fail to do so in others. The dosage of the interacting drug may be an important factor. A small dose of H_2 antagonist cimetidine may fail to inhibit the metabolism of the anticoagulant drug warfarin. However, a large dose may have great clinical effects. Sometimes, the interactions can be avoided using another member of the same group of drugs. Doxycycline level in serum can fall below therapeutic concentration if phenytoin, barbiturates or carbamazepine are given concurrently, but tetracyclins do not affect in the same manner. Some doctors are over-anxious about drug interaction and other clinicians virtually disregard the existance of drug interactions. The responsible position lies between these two extremes. A good number of interacting drugs can be given together safely if proper precaution is taken.

Today, polypharmacy is the norm rather than an exception and there is enormous potential for drug interactions in the patients. Estimates of the incidence of Drug-Drug interactions have been reported in as high as 20% of patients who are on more than 5 medications at a time. Awareness of potential of drug interaction is essential for a practicing physician to enable the patient to receive the best medical care that he is entitled to.

A drug interaction refers to the possibility that one drug may alter the pharmacological effect of another drug given concurrently. The net result may be enhanced or diminished effect of one or both of the drugs or a new effect that is not seen with either drug alone. Drug interaction is particularly important for those drugs with narrow therapeutic index, where even small elevations in plasma concentration can cause potentially serious adverse reaction.

There are two main types of drug interactions.

Pharmacokinetic interactions occur when one drug affects the plasma concentration or half-life or both of another by altering its absorption, distribution, metabolism or elimination. Example includes competition for protein binding in the plasma and alteration of hepatic cytocrome P450.

Pharmacodynamic interactions occur when one drug affects the ability of another to bring about its effects. This might occur with drugs that bind to multiple receptor types. Or it may even occur with the inadvertent concomitant use of mutually antagonistic agents such as β-agonists for bronchial asthma.

Drug interaction can be largely predicted on the pharmacological properties of the drugs being co-administered. A large number of drugs are metabolized (inactivated) by the hepatic microsomal cytochrome P450 enzymes. Some examples of drugs (with narrow therapeutic index) being metabolized by these enzymes includes:

- Non-sedating antihistamines
- Long acting opiate analgesics
- Antiarrythmics
- Long acting benzodiazepines
- Ergotamines and dihydroergotamine
- Illicit drugs
- Coumarin anticoagulants
- Oral Contraceptives

A number of drugs also alter the functioning of these enzymes. Some examples include:

Cytochrome P450 inhibitors

- HIV protease inhibitors
- Non-nucleoside reverse transcriptase inhibitors
- Macrolide antibiotics
- Azole antifungal
- Cimetidine

Cytochrome P450 inducers

- HIV protease inhibitors
- Non-nucleoside reverse transcriptase inhibitors
- Anticonvulsants (that are P450 inducers)

Co-administration of drugs having a narrow therapeutic index with either inducers or inhibitors of the cytochrome P450 enzymes could lead to either therapeutic failure or toxicity.

Similarly, drug interactions are also particularly relevant for antibiotics, which are amongst the commonest group of drugs prescribed. Many interactions take place at the absorption stage. Antacids and antidiarrhoeal preparations, in particular, can delay and reduce the absorption of anti-biotics such as tetracycline and clindamycin, by combining with them in the gastro-intestinal tract to form chelates or complexes. The potentiation of toxic side effects of one drug by another is a common type of interaction. Antibiotics, which are implicated in this type of interaction, are those, which themselves possess some toxicity such as aminoglycosides, some cephalosporins, tetracyclines and colistin. Some of the most important adverse interactions with antibiotics are those which involve other drugs which have a low toxicity/efficacy ratio. These include warfarin; phenytoin and tolbutamide. Co-administration of antibacterial drugs such as penicillin whose efficacy is dependent on bacterial cell division along with bacteriostatic drugs such as tetracycline would lead to significant reduced efficacy of the former.

Thus, one can easily appreciate the importance of awareness regarding drug interactions to avoid iatrogenic adverse effects and therapeutic failure.

Outside the Body Interactions

Sometimes, some drugs are added to infusion fluid to achieve better clinical effects. There is change for incompatibility between the drugs and the infusion fluid. Effect of soluble insulin can be reduced if it is drawn up with potassium zinc insulin in the same syringe or drip. If diazepam is added to infusion fluid, precipitation reaction will be caused.

Factors Contributing to the Occurance of Drug Interaction

The number of factors contributing to drug interaction is listed below:

1. **Multiple pharmacological effects:** A single drug affects many physiologic systems and so concurrent administration of another drug can also affect the same system. In these conditions normally the primary action of the drug is focused out looking the secondary action. Example: a combined therapy of phenothiazine

antipsychotic (eg, chlorpromazine) and a tricyclic antidepressant (eg, trihexyphenidyl) is employed frequently. Both have their specific primary actions and also have slight anticholinergic effect which however becomes a significant additive effect.

2. **Multiple prescribers:** Most commonly an individual visits a family doctor along with other specialist (eg, dentist, cardiologist) leading to multiple prescribers for the same patient where each prescriber is unaware of the medication prescribed by the other. Example: One physician may prescribe an antihistamine for a patient for whom another physician has prescribed an antianxiety agent, with the possible consequence of an excessive depressant effect.

3. **Use of non-prescription drugs:** It involves the concurrent administration of a prescription drug with a non-prescription drug (eg, antacids, asparin) and even sometimes concurrent administration of two or more non-prescription drugs. In some situations two non-prescription drugs may contain the same active ingredient(s) leading to additive effects.

4. **Patient noncompliance:** Either lack of or improper or confusion in instruction from a patient or pharmacist may lead to noncompliance for patients. Also many patients donot take medication in the manner intended by the prescriber. Example: Some patient if he forgets a dose doubles the next dose to make for it.

5. **Drug abuse:** The tendencies of some individuals to abuse or deliberately misuse drugs also may lead to an increased incidence of drug interactions. Example includes the abusive use of barbiturates, narcotic analgesics, etc.

The severity of a drug interaction is difficult to predict as there are many variables governing it. Some of these variables include dosage, route of administration, time of administration, sequence of administration and duration of therapy. The other variables are related to patient and are briefly listed below:

(i) **Age:** Studies indicated that there is an increased incidence of adverse drug reactions and drug interaction in both young and geriatric patients. Among the young the drug related interaction frequently occurs in infants as they donot have fully developed enzyme systems for the metabolism of certain drugs and also have immature renal function. Geriatric patients most frequently experience one or more disease states like renal failure leading to alteration in drug response. Also with age there are changes in the absorption, distribution, metabolism and excretion of drugs leading to increased incidence of both adverse drug reactions and drug interactions.

(ii) **Genetic factors:** It leads to the development of an unexpected drug response in a particular patient. Example: Isoniazid is metabolized by an acetylation process, the rate of which is under genetic control. Therefore, some patients taking isoniazid suffer from peripheral neuritis as they are slow acetylators.

(iii) **Disease states:** Occurrence of a one or more disease along with the disease for which the particular drug is prescribed may influence patients' response to a drug. Example: Many drugs are bound extensively to plasma proteins and only the unbound fraction of the drug is active. So any reduction in the amount of protein consequently alters the availability of the drug and also its activity.

(iv) **Renal function:** For drugs which are primarily excreted from the liver in its active form are administered for a prolonged period to a renal impaired patient which may lead to an increased and prolonged effect of the drug. Therefore the dosage of the drug must be carefully adjusted and also caution must be taken for concurrent administration of potentially interacting drugs.

(v) **Hepatic failure:** Many drugs get metabolized in the liver. Therefore impairment in hepatic function may lead to prolongation of drug effect. Also some drugs get metabolized by liver enzymes. Therefore concurrent administration of drugs affecting the particular enzyme may also affect in drug metabolism. Example: Drugs like barbiturates are known to stimulate the activity of liver enzymes (enzyme induction). It may lead to rapid metabolism and excretion of concurrently administered agents which are metabolized by these enzymes.

(vi) **Alcohol consumption:** Chronic use of alcoholic beverages may increase the rate of metabolism of drugs such as warfarin, phenytoin and tolbutamide probably by increasing the activity of liver enzymes. Also concurrent use of alcoholic beverages with sedatives and other depressant drugs could result in an excessive depression.

(vii) **Smoking:** The activity of drug-metabolizing liver enzymes also gets affected by smoking according to some studies. Example: diazepam, theophylline, etc. This effect is more pronounced in young and middle-aged individuals.

(viii) **Diet:** Concurrent administration of food and drug may affect the absorption of drug from gastrointestinal tract. For example, many penicillin and tetracycline derivative must be given atleast 1 hour before or 2 hours after the meal for optimal absorption.

(ix) **Environmental factors:** Chemicals in the environment such as DDT may increase the activity of liver enzymes leading to increase in rate of metabolism of certain drugs.

(x) **Individual variation:** Wide variety of variation is present in response to a particular drug. Example: plasma levels of tricyclic anti-depressants vary widely among individuals using the same dosage regimen over the same time period.

Mechanism of Drug Interactions

The mechanism of drug interaction can be subdivided into two types;

(a) Pharmacokinetic Interactions and

(b) Pharmacodynamic Interactions.

(a) Pharmacokinetic Interactions

It is the interaction in which the process of drugs absorption (A), distribution (D), biotransformation (metabolization) (M) and excretion (E) [ADME processes] are altered affecting the desired drug action.

Interaction during Absorption

The majority of the drugs are orally given for absorption through the gastrointestinal tract. Resultantly, interaction within the gut will certainly alter the absorption pattern of the drugs. There are some drugs which are given chronically (e.g. oral anticoagulants) to the patients. In that case, total amount of drug absorption is important so that it should not be altered markedly. Besides there are drugs (e.g. hypnotics and analgesics) which are given as single doses. In this case absorption should be rapid; reduction of the absorption rate may cause failure to secure adequate serum levels.

Effect of the gastrointestinal pH changes: Absorption of a drug from gastrointestinal tract depends on the pKa value of the drug. Higher the non-ionized form (lipid soluble form) higher is the rate of drug absorption from the GI tract. The absorption of salicylic acid from the stomach is much higher at low pH (more unionized form) than at high pH. So, alteration of gastric pH may alter the absorption of the drug.

Adsorption, chelation and other complex mechanisms: Activated charcoal is used as an adsorbing agent who can adsorb drugs within the gut to hinder proper absorption of the drugs from GI tract. Antacids can also adsorb a good number of drugs. Tetracyclin can chelate with di and tri-valent metallic ions such as aluminum, bismuth, calcium, iron etc., so, absorption of antibiotic will be reduced. Antacids and milk can also reduce the absorption of tetracyclin from the gut. This type of interaction can be minimized by administering the two (tetracyclin + antacid or milk) at 2-3 hrs interval. Alteration of the gut flora by antibiotics may disrupt the enterohepatic cycling of oral contraceptives and digoxin. Cholestyramine (amonic exchange resin) binds to a considerable number of drugs if co-administered (e.g. digoxin, warfarin, thyroxine) and can reduce their absorption.

Altering gastrointestinal motility: Alteration of gastrointestinal tract motility may influence the rate of drug absorption. Most of the drugs are absorbed from upper part of small intestine. There are some drugs, which can alter the rate of stomach emptying thereby altering the absorption of drugs. Anticholinergic drugs and metoclopramide decrease or increase gastrointestinal motility respectively and can alter the bio-availability of many drugs. Tricyclic antidepressants increase the absorption of dicumarol because they increase the time available for dissolution and absorption. On the other hand, in case of levodopa they reduce the absorption by increasing the intestinal mucosal metabolism of levodopa. Pethidine and diamorphine can reduce the absorption of other drugs from gastrointestinal tract.

Malabsorption caused by drugs: The antibiotic neomycin may cause impairment of a number of drugs like Digoxin, PenicillinV, etc.

Interaction during Distribution

Displacement from plasma protein binding sites: Some drugs during distribution in circulation can bind with plasma proteins, particularly albumins. There are drugs, which bind extremely with plasma protein. The drug dicomarol has only out of every 1000 molecules remain free at serum concentration of 0.5mg per 100 mL. Digoxin can bind to the muscle of heart to exert its pharmacological effects. The drug, which is greatly bound to albumin, can be displaced from its binding site by another drug which has greater affinity for the same binding site. The displaced (and now active) drug molecules come to the plasma water where its concentration rapidly rises. Drugs like aspirin competes with anticoagulant drug warfarin for same protein binding site thereby, the concentration of displaced warfarin will be high with increased adverse effects. The major metabolite of chloral hydrate is trichloroacetic acid which can displace warfarin, thereby increasing anticoagulant effects. Only drugs with low apparent volume of distribution (V_d) will be affected by this type of displacement phenomenon. Such drugs include tolbutamide (96% bound, V_d 101) and oral anticoagulants such as warfarin (99% bound, V_d 91) and phenytoin (90% bound, V_d 351)

Displacement from other tissue binding sites: Quinidine can displace digoxin from binding sites in the tissues. So, when a patient is given quinidine who is receiving digoxin, the concentration of digoxin will greatly increase pharmacological effects.

Interaction during Biotransformation

A large number of drugs are metabolized (biotransformed) inside the body to move water soluble forms for easy excretion from kidney. If this process (biotransformation) was not so, many drugs would remain in the body for a long period and pharmacological effects would also be continued. Most of this biotransformation is carried out by these enzymes of liver cells. Some drugs are also metabolized in the serum, kidneys, the skin and the intestine.

Induction of enzymes: Enzyme induction by drugs can enhance metabolism of drugs and the therapeutic achievement will be less. Barbiturates increase the enzyme activities with increased metabolism and excretion. So, tolerance can develop with the repeated use of barbiturates.

If a drug D1 is biotransformed by the enzymes, then concurrent dosing of another drug D2 which can induce the same enzyme system can enhance the metabolism of drug D1. Anticoagulant activity of the drug warfarin can be decreased with the concurrent administration of enzyme inducing agent, dichloralphenazone. Enzyme induction is a very common mechanism of interaction. This type of interaction can also be caused by chlorinated hydrocarbon insecticides such as dichlophane and lindane. Tobacco smoking also acts as enzyme inducer.

Phase1 oxidation is a metabolic pathway which is commonly affected by enzyme induction. Phase1 oxidation covers a number of metabolic biotransformations, all of which require the presence of NADPH and P450. At the time of enzyme induction, endoplasmic reticulum amount of liver cells increases and cytochrome P450 level also rises.

Enzymes inhibition: There are other drugs which can act as enzyme inhibitors and potentiate the action of other drugs whose pharmacological actions are limited by being metabolized. If an epileptic patient, who is dependent on phenytoin is given chloramphenicol (enzyme inhibitor) concurrently, the phenytoin level in blood may increase with possible toxicity. Metabolism of anticoagulant drug is increased by cimetidine. So, there is a change of excess warfarin accumulation with hemorrhage. Clinical significance of this type of enzyme inhibition depends on the increase of serum level of drugs. If this level remains within therapeutic concentration, the enzyme inhibition may be advantageous. If serum level of drug rises to the toxic range due to inhibitor drug, then interaction becomes adverse.

Alteration of blood flow through liver: Orally absorbed drugs enter the liver by portal circulation before they are distributed throughout the body for pharmacological effects. This phenomenon is called first pass. During this first pass a substantial number of fat soluble drugs undergo biotransformation. Some concurrently administered drugs can influence this first pass metabolism. For example, H_2 antagonist cimetidine can reduce hepatic blood flow and thereby increase bioavailability of propranolol. A number of other drugs have opposite effect with increment of hepatic flow so that their biotransformation is increased.

Interaction during Excretion

Most of the drugs (exception: Inhalation anaesthetics) are excreted via bile or urine. The blood passes to the kidney tubules where drugs and their matabolites are removed from blood by active-energy transport system. This removed drugs along with metabolites are deposited into the tubular filtrate. The tubular cells also possess active or passive transport system for reabsorption of drugs and metabolites. So, any action by drugs, with kidney tubules fluid pH, with active transport systems and with blood flow to kidney can alter the rate of excretion of other drugs and metabolites. For example, the drug probenecid interferes with penicillin for active transport process at the kidney and thereby prolongs the action of penicillins. This effect is pharmacologically beneficial.

Changes in urinary pH and drug interactions: Any alteration of urinary pH influence ionization of drugs and its excretion. Only the un-ionized form of the drug is lipid soluble and can diffuse back through the lipid membrane of tubule cells. Hence, at high pH value (alkaline range) weakly acidic drugs with low pH value (3.0-7.5) will remain in ionized stage (lipid insoluble stage) and therefore pass through urine. Enhance excretion of absorption (acidic drug) occurs if sodium bicarbonate is given (alkaline pH). Similarly, weak organic bases (pKa value of 7.5-10.5) at low pH range (acidic) will be excreted via urine rapidly. The basic drug amphetamine will be rapidly excreted if ammonium chloride is given.

Clinically, significance of this phenomenon is largely metabolized in liver and a few drugs are excreted in urine in unchanged form. In case of overdosage, pH of urine is changed deliberately to increase the drug loss via urine. Example: phenobarbitone and salicylates.

Interaction due to kidney blood flow: Prostaglandins present in kidney act as vasodialator and blood flow through kidney partially depends on it. Indomethacin can inhibit the prostaglandin synthesis and serum excretion of lithium is reduced. Therefore, serum level of lithium will be high.

Interactions due to biliary secretion and enterohepatic shunt: Some drugs are excreted to bile in unchanged or conjugated form (as glucosonide to make them water soluble). Intestinal flora can change some conjugated drugs to parent drugs and these are then reabsorbed. The reabsorption process will help to prolong the stay of drugs inside the body. An antibiotic can affect this gut flora and recycling process of some drugs can be affected.

Possible sites of Drug Interaction

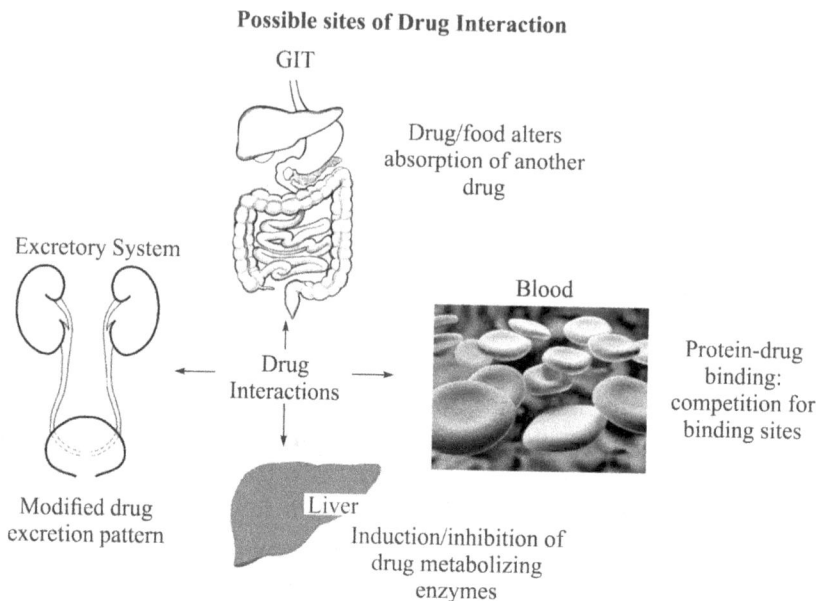

GIT

Drug/food alters absorption of another drug

Excretory System

Blood

Protein-drug binding: competition for binding sites

Drug Interactions

Modified drug excretion pattern

Liver
Induction/inhibition of drug metabolizing enzymes

(b) Pharmacodynamic Interactions

Sometimes a patient can take two or more drugs at the same time. Pharmacodynamic interaction may happen in this case. The effects of one drug if changed by the presence of another drug at the site of action, is called pharmacodynamic drug interaction. The use of two or more drugs can induce no effect, synergism or antagonism.

Drug antagonism or opposing interaction: When the effect of a drug is reduced or abolished by the presence of another drug, then it can be termed antagonism. Drug antagonism can be classified into three types:

(i)   Chemical antagonism

(ii) Physiological antagonism and

(iii) Pharmacological antagonism

(i)   *Chemical antagonism:* When a simple chemical reaction is involved between two drugs and effect of one drug is reduced or abolished then it is called chemical antagonism. For example, non-absorbable antacids neutralize the gastric acid;

(ii) *Physiological antagonism:* Physiological antagonism is that when physiological effect of a drug is antagonized by drug acting on two different types of receptors. Acetylcholine contracts smooth muscle of intestine through muscarinic cholinoceptors. But this action is antagonized by adrenaline via adrenoceptors;

(iii) *Pharmacological antagonism:* When a drug action is antagonized by other drug via same receptor, then it is called pharmacological antagonism. This is of two types:

(i) Competitive,

(ii) Non-competitive.

(i) **Competitive antagonism:** When two drugs compete for the same receptor and antagonism happens then it can be termed competitive antagonism. This type of antagonism is reversible. Acetylcholine can contract intestinal smooth muscle and this effect can be competitively antagonized by atropine.

(ii) **Non-competitive antagonism:** When maximum response of an antagonist is reduced in presence of antagonist, then this is called non-competitive antagonism.

Drug synergism: When two drugs with same pharmacological effect are given together the effect can be additive. This type of phenomenon is called drug synergism. It is of two types:

(i) Additive effect

(ii) Potentiation effect.

(i) **Additive effect:** When two drugs are used together and the effect is equal to the sum of individual effects then it is called additive effect. For example, alcohol in moderate amounts with other hypnotics or tranquillizers may produce excessive depression of central nervous system. Additive effects can occur with therapeutic or toxic effects of two drugs. Sometimes the additive effects are solely toxic. (e.g. additive toxicity, nephrotoxicity or bone marrow depression)

(ii) **Potentiation effect:** When the effect of two drugs concurrently used is greater than the sum of the individual drug effects the effect is called potentiation. For example, combination of two antimicrobials like sulphamethoxazole and trimethoprim can produce potentiation.

Alteration of drug transport mechanism and drug interactions: There are some drugs which can prevent other drugs to reach adrenergic neurones for action. The drugs like tricyclic antidepressants prevent the re-uptake of noradrenaline into peripheral adrenergic neurones so that its effects are increased. The tricyclic antidepressants are also able to prevent the uptake of clonidine within CNS and therefore, its antihypertensive effects are blocked.

Disturbances in fluid and electrolyte balance and cause of drug interaction: Sometimes, any change of fluid and electrolytes can cause pharmacodynamic interactions. For example, the antidiuretic drug frusemide depletes potassium in urine and plasma concentration may fall with increasing sensitivity and toxicity of digitalis glycoside. Thiazide diuretics can alter the sodium excretion via kidney which may cause decrease in excretion of lithium and lithium concentration of plasma will rise.

Drug Interactions Tables

Alcohols[1]

Drugs	Interaction with	Effects
Alcohol	**Antihistamines** (a) Promethazine, chlorpheniramine, dyphenylhydramines. (b) Astimizole, loralidine terfenadine	(a) Additive CNS depression action. (b) Minimal or absence of additive effect.
	Aspirin	Prolongation of bleeding time can be increased.
	Atropine	Marked impairment of attention found.
	Barbiturates	Additive CNS depression.
	Benzodiazepines	CNS depressant action of benzodiazepines and alcohol are additive.
	Bromvaletone or Ethinamate	Additive CNS depressant action.
	Buspirone	Additive alcohol action.
	Butyraldoxime	Disulfiram action.
	Caffeine	No counteract effect found
	Calcium channel blockers	Blood alcohol level increased
	Cephalosporin antibiotics	Disulphiram like action.
	Chloral hydrate	Additive CNS depressant action.
	Cimetidine, Famotidine, Ranitidine	Additive CNS depressant action.
	CNS depressants	Additive action.
	Codeine	No interaction with small amount of codeine but additive reaction with higher doses.
	Dextropropoxyphene	Additive CNS depressant action.
	Dimethylformamide	Disulfiram like reaction.
	Disulfiram	Flushlessness and fullness of face and neck, trachycardia, breathlessness, giddiness and hypotension, nausea and vomiting.
	Fluoxetine, Femoxetine	No effects.
	Fluvoxamine	Additive effects.
	Clovaxamine	No effects.
	Glutethimide	Additive reaction, psychomotor skill is impaired.
	Glyceryl trinitrate	Faint and dizziness may arise.
	Griseofulvin	The intoxicant effects of alcohol may increase.
	Hydromophine	Additive CNS depressant action.
	Indomethacin or Phenylbutazone	Additive action of alcohol.

Contd...

Drugs	Interaction with	Effects
	Isoniazid	Additive action.
	Ketoconazole	Disulfiram like reaction may occur.
	Lithium carbonate	Additive action.
	Maprotiline	Additive action.
	Meprobamate	The intoxicant effects can be increased.
	Methaqualone or *Mandrax* (methaqualone + diphenhydramine)	Additive CNS depressant action.
	Metoclopramide	Sedative effects may increase.
	Metronidazole	Disulfiram like reaction.
	Nitrofurantoin	No firm interaction found.
	Nitroimidazoles	Disulfiram like reaction.
	Paraldehyde	Additive CNS depressant action. (in the treatment of acute intoxication fatal effects results)
	Phenothiazines, Butyrophenones and other drugs	Additive effects
	Procarbazine	Flushing reaction.
	Sodium cromoglycate	No adverse interaction
	Tetracyclic antidepressant (a) Mianserin (b) Pirlindole	(a) additive action (b) no interaction
	Tolazoline	Disulfiram like reaction may appear.
	Trazodone	Additive action.
	Trichloroethylene	A flushing skin reaction similar to a mild disulfiram reaction.
	Tricyclic antidepressant (a) Amitriptylene (b) Doxepin (c) Nortriptylene, Clomipramine, Desipramine, amoxapine	(a) Impairment is increased. (b) Impairment is increased. (c) Only minimal interaction.
	Viqualine	No adverse interaction.
	Xylene	Dizziness and nausea, and a flushing skin reaction.
	Food (a) Edible fungi *Coprinus atramentarius, Boletus luridus* and others. (b) Milk	(a) Disulfiram like reaction. (b) Blood level of alcohol and its intoxicant effects will be reduced.

Analgesic & Non - Steroidal Anti - inflammatory Drugs[1, 2]

Drugs	Interaction with	Effects
Alfentanil	Erythromycin	Prolonged and increased alfentanil effects.
Antirheumatic agents (indomethacin, salicylates etc.)	Mazindol	No adverse affects
Aspirin & Salicylates	Carbonic anhydrase	In high dose fatality may arise.
	Cimetidine or Ranitidine	Negligible clinical effect with cimetidine but no interaction with ranitidine.
	Corticosteroids	Gastrointestinal bleeding and ulceration may be increased.
	Levamisole	No effects confirmed yet.
	Methotrexate	Effect potentiate.
	Phenylbutazone	Reduces uricosuric effects by aspirin.
	Phenytoin	Level will increase.
	Probenecid	Mutually antagonists
	Sulphinpyrazone	Mutually antagonists
	Spironolactone	Antagonistic action.
Azapropazone	Miscellaneous drugs	No significant effect
Buprenorphine	Amitriptyline	Potentiation with alcohol, other CNS depressant and MOls Diazepam may produce respiratory and cardiac collaps.
Dextromoramide	Triacetyloleandomycin	An isolated report describes marked increase of dextromoramide and coma.
Dextropropoxyphene	Orphenadrine	Potentiation with alcohol, CNS depressant, decrease efficacy of heavy smokers.
	Tobacco smoking	Analgesic effect of the drug is less in those who smoke.
Diclofenac	Miscellaneous drugs	Increase blood level of lithium and digoxin, inhibit diuretics but potentiate sparing diuretics. Increase toxicity of methotrexate lowers serum level of salicylates.

Contd...

Drugs	Interaction with	Effects
Diflunisal	Non steroidal anti-inflammatory agents and analgesics (a) Aspirin (b) Indomethacin (c) Paracetamol & Naproxen	(a) Reduce the serum diflunisal levels (b) Serum Indomethacin level raises 2-3 folds (c) Paracetamol levels are increased but not those of naproxen.
Flufenamic, Mefenamic and Tolfenamic acids, Oxyphenbutazone or Phenylbutazone.	Antacids	Absorption of fenamates is accelerated by magnesium hydroxide but retarded by aluminum hydroxide. Sodium bicarbonate shows no effect.
Flufenamic or Mefenamic acid	Cholestyramine	Absorption of both is reduced.
Ibuprofen	Antacids	Aspirin displaces ibuprophen from serum binding sites hence should be avoided.
	Aspirin	Methotrexate and lithium toxicity may increase. Antagonises the effect of frusemide & thiazides. Anticoagulants may increase the risk of GI ulceration.
Ibuprofen or Flurbiprofen	Cimetidine, Nizatidine or Ranitidine.	Frusimides effects reduces, aspirin reduces serum level of Flurbiprofen. Digoxin absorption may be delayed. Anticoagulants effects may be interfered.
Indomethacin	Allopurinol	Alcohol and smoking associated with increased risk of peptic ulceration. Diflunisal may cause fatal GI haemorrhage in susceptible individuals. Anticoagulants may cause severe GI ulcers.
	Antacids	Irritation of the gut caused by indomethacin can be reduced by antacids.
	Aspirin and salicylates	No significant effect.

Contd...

Drugs	Interaction with	Effects
	Cimetidine	Cause small reduction in the serum level of indomethacin without anti-inflammatory effects being altered.
	Probenecid	Serum indomethacin level can be doubled causing improvement in arthritis patients but toxicity may occur prominently in those whose kidney function is impaired.
	Vaccines	Limited evidence suggests more severe effect.
Isoxicam	Miscellaneous drugs	Blood loss is increased.
Vetoprofen	Probenecid	May reduce loss from the body and increase its serum level. Increased toxicity is a possibility.
Meclofenamic acid	Aspirin	Intestinal bleeding is increased by concurrent use.
	Anti –convulsants	Reduce methadone effect.
	Disulfiram	No adverse affect
Methadone	Rifampicin (rifampin)	Reduction in serum level.
	Urinary acidifers or alkalizers	If the urine is made acidic, increment is observed from the body and if is made alkaline, reduction occurs.
Morphine	Cimetidine or Ranitidine	Isolated reports describe disorientation, confusion and agitation in a patient taking morphine and ranitidine. Other CNS depressants, alcohol, muscle relaxants, MAO inhibitor potentiate effect and cause respiratory depression. Diuretics antagonise morphine effect. Analgesic effects are potentiated with NSAID's.
	Contraceptives [oral]	The clearance of morphine is nearly doubled by concurrent use of the oral contraceptives.
	Metoclopramide	Increases the rate of absorption of oral morphine and enhance its sedative effects.

Contd...

Drugs	Interaction with	Effects
Nabumetone	Tricyclic antidepressants	The bioavailability and the degree of analgesia are increased by the concurrent use.
	Antacids	Absorption can be altered using antacids with uncertain clinical importance.
	Aspirin and Salicylates	Serum naproxen levels may be increased or reduced without clinical effectiveness being disturbed.
Naproxen	Cholestyramine	Enhances the effect of oral anticoagulants, phenytoin, methotrexate, sulphonamides, sulphonylurea, hypoglycaemics. Diuretics increase risk of renal disorders. Absorption reduced by antacids and increased by bicarbonates.
	Cimetidine	Does not affect.
	Probenacids	Serum levels are raised by 50% with probably minimum clinical importance.
Narcotic analgesics	Sulglycotide	Does not affect.
	Benzodiazepines	Having potent sedative effects of opiates appear to be opposed.
	Promethazone	Having potent sedative effects, would be expected to be additive with CNS depressant effects.
Nefopam	Miscellaneous drugs	Should avoid taking anticonvulsants or the MAOI. Side effects are somewhat increased. Concurrent use of tricyclic antidepressants may result in exagerated antimuscaric effects such as blurred vision, dry mouth, urinary retention.

Contd...

Drugs	Interaction with	Effects
Oxyphenylbutazone and Phenylbutazone	Antacids	No significant change in absorption rate except ketoprofen where a small reduction can occur.
	Sucralfate	Does not interact adversely and also possibly protect the gastric mucosa from damage.
	Anabolic steroids	Serum oxyphenylbutazone levels are increased by 40%. Phenylbutazone appears to be unaffected.
Paracetamol (Acetaminophen)	Alcohol	Severe liver damage, fatal in some instances, who take moderate doses of paracetamol. Enhances anti-coagulant activities. Absorption of paracetamol is reduced by pethidine and propantheline.
	Anticholinergic agents	Delays gastric emptying
	Barbiturates	Hepatotoxicity developed in a woman.
	Cholestyramine	Absorption may be reduced if both taken at a time but if cholestyramine is given in a hour later, very little reduction in absorption.
	Cimetidine	No interaction of clinical importance.
Paracetamol and other drugs	Opiate analgesics	Morphine and diamorphine delay gastric emptying causing reduced rate of other drugs.
Paracetamol	Oral contraceptives	Cleared from the body move quickly in woman taking oral contraceptives. Paracetamol increases the absorption of ethinyloestradiol from the gut by about 20%.
D-Penicillamine	Antacids	Absorption can be reduced by 30-40% by antacids containing aluminum and magnesium hydroxides are taken concurrently.

Contd...

Drugs	Interaction with	Effects
Pentazocine	Iron Preparations	Can reduce as much as two thirds by the concurrent use.
	Tobacco smoking and environmental pollution.	Those who smoke or urban dwellers require 50% or more for satisfactory analgesia than those who don't smoke or live where the air is clean. Respiratory depression effect with halothane, Iidocaine.
Pethidine (Meperidine)	Acyclovir	CNS depression effect is potentiated by alcohol and other CNS depressants. Hydroxyzine enhances analgesic effects.
Pethidine	Chlopromazine and other phenothiazines.	An isolated report describes toxicity.
	Cimetidine or Ranitidine	Increased respiratory depression, sedation, CNS toxicity and hypotension can occur if used together.
Pethidine (Meperidine)	Furazolidine	Hyperpyrexic reaction may occur on concurrent use in man which is yet to be confirmed.
	Monoamine oxidase inhibitors (MAOI).	May result in life threatening reaction in a few patients. Excitement, muscle rigidity, hyperpyrexia, flushing sweating occurs rapidly. Respiratory depression, hypotension may occur.
	Phenytoin	May reduce serum levels and increase toxic metabolite, clinical importance yet to be confirmed.
Phenazone (Antipyrine)	Miscellaneous drugs	Changes in the half life.
Phenoperidine	Antacids	An antacid showed the increase in the serum level.
	Beta-blockers	An isolated report describes a patient with tetanus showing fall in blood pressure.

Contd...

Drugs	Interaction with	Effects
	Allopurinol	No significant interaction.
	Barbiturates	No report having clinical importance.
	Indomethacin	An isolated report describes an insignificant deterioration in renal function.
	Methyl phenidate	May increase serum level.
	Pesticides	May increase the rate of metabolism.
	Tobacco smoking	The loss from the body is greater in smokers than in non-smokers.
Phenylbutazone or Oxyphenylbutazone	Tricyclic antidepressants	Can delay the absorption from the gut.
Piroxicam and Tenoxicam	Cholestyramine	May increase the loss of both from the body leading to loss by their therapeutic effects accordingly.
Piroxicam	Cimetidine	No significant interaction.
Sulindac	Dimethylsulfoxide (DMSO)	A single report describes serious peripheral neuropathy when applied on skin.

Antiarrythmic[1, 2]

Drugs	Interaction with	Effects
Ajmaline	Lignocaine (Lidocaine) or Quinidine	An isolated report describes cardiac failure in a patient administered concurrently.
Amiodarone	Anaesthetics	Risk of complication and death increased.
	Beta-blockers	Brabicardia, venticular fibrillation and asystole are reported on abdominal application.
	Calcium channel blockers	Sinus arrest and serious hypotension occurs.
	Cholestyramine	Reduce absorption.
	Cimetidine	Causes rise in the serum level.
	Disopyramide, Propafenone or Mexiletine	The risk of atypical ventricular trachycardia or effect seems to be increased.

Contd...

Drugs	Interaction with	Effects
Apridine	Amiodarone	Serum levels may be increased.
Disopyramide or procainamide	Antacids	Inconclusive evidence suggests that aluminum containing antacids may cause a small reduction in absorption.
Disopyramide	Anticholinergic	The effect may be expected to be additive.
	Beta-blockers	Adverse interactions between these drugs may be uncommon.
	Erythromycin	Cardiac arrythmias may occur.
	Phenobarbitone	Levels in the serum are reduced on concurrent use.
	Phenytion	Levels in the serum may be reduced on concurrent use and may fall below therapeutic concentration. Loss of arrythmia may occur.
	Quinidine	May be raised slightly.
Disopyramide	Rifampicin	May cause marked reduction in serum levels on concurrent use.
Encainide	Diltiazem	May cause sharp increase in serum levels with the slight increase of active metabolites
	Miscellaneous drugs	No interaction having clinical significance is reported except the effect of cimetidine which should be monitored.
	Quinidine	May cause a marked reduction in the clearance of encainide in those who are extensive metaboliser of encainide.
Flecainide	Amiodarone	Serum levels are increased.
	Cholestyramine	An isolated report describes reduced serum levels.
	Cimetidine	May increase serum levels.
	Food or antacids	Absorption is not significantly altered in adults but may possibly be reduced by milk in infants.
	Quinine	Reduce the metabolism.
	Tobacco smoking	Tobacco smokers need larger doses.

Contd...

Drugs	Interaction with	Effects
Lignocaine (Lidocine)	Beta blockers	Serum level may be increased.
	Cimetidine	Reduces the clearness of lignocaine and raises serum levels. Toxicity may occur if dosage is not reduced. Ranitidine appears to interact minimally.
Lignocaine (Lidocaine)	Disopyramide	No report having clinical justification is known.
	Morphine	No significant effect.
	Phynitoin	Central toxic side effects may be increased on concurrent intravenous infusion. Serum levels are slightly reduced but markedly reduced if given orally.
	Procainamide	An isolated case of delirium is reported.
	Tocainide	Toxic chronic Seizure in a man is reported.
Lorcainide	Rifampicin	Massed reduction in serum levels and failure to central ventricular tachycardia in a man is reported.
Mexiletine	Antacids, Urinary acidifiers and alkalinizers.	No remarkable effect.
	Antiarrythmic drugs	Concurrent use is reported to be beneficial with reduced side effects.
	Cimetidine or Ranitidine	No adverse interaction on concurrent administration.
	Diamorphine or Morphine	Absorption may be repressed in patients following a myocardial infraction and depression is marked and delayed if used concurrently.
	Phenytoin	Serum levels may be reduced on concurrent use.
	Rifampicin (Rifampin)	The clearness from the body is increased on concurrent use causing the need of increased dosage.
Moricizine (Ethomozine)	Cimetidine	Increases the serum levels.

Contd…

Drugs	Interaction with	Effects
Pirmental	Rifampicin (Rifampin)	Increases the loss from the body, then reduces the antirrythmic effect.
Procainamide	Amiodarone	Serum levels are increased by about 60% and used concurrently. Reduction in dosage is required to avoid toxicity.
	Beta blockers	Pharmacokinetics are widely changed.
	Cimetidine or Ranitidine	Serum level may be increased on concurrent application and toxicity may develop precisely to those having reduced renal clearance. Ranitidine appears not to interact significantly.
	Para-aminobenzoic acid (PABA)	A single report describes the reduction in metabolism by increasing serum levels.
	Quinidine	A single report describes marked increase in serum levels on concurrent use.
	Trimethoprin	Causes marked increase in serum levels.
Propafenone	Cimetidine	No adverse interaction.
	Miscellaneous drugs	May oppose the effects of others. Shortness of breath and a worsening of the control of asthma is reported.
	Quinidine	It doubles the serum levels.
Quinidine	Amiodarone	Serum levels may be approximately doubled on concurrent administration. Reduction in dosage is advised to avoid toxicity and the risk of a typical ventricular tachycardia.
Quinidine	Anticonvulsants	Serum levels may be reduced on concurrent use. Loss of arrhythmia control is possible if quinidine dosage is not increased.
	Aspirin	A patient showed a two to three fold increase in bleeding times.

Contd...

Drugs	Interaction with	Effects
	Beta blockers	Normally an advantageous interaction.
	Calcium Channel Blockers	Depression in serum levels are reported on concurrent use of nifidipine and which doubled on being withdrawn. Diltia Zem does not interact.
	Cimetidine and Ranitidine	Serum levels may rise and intoxication may develop on concurrent use. An isolated report describes ventricular bigenuiy when ranitidine was used.
	Kaolin-Pectin	Can reduce the absorption and reduce serum levels.
	Ketoconazol	Describes marked increase in serum levels in man.
	Laxatives	Serum level may reduce on concurrent use.
	Lignocaine (Lidocaine)	A single report describes sinoartrial arreston concurrent use.
	Metoclopramide	May reduce the absorption from a sustained released formulation but may increase the absorption with other preparations.
	Rifampicine (Rifarnpin)	Serum levels and its therapeutic effects may be markedly reduced by the concurrent use.
Quinidine	Urinary alkalinizer and antacids	Large rise in the urinary pH due to concurrent use can cause the retention, which may lead to intoxication.
Tocainide	Urinary alkalinizer and antacids	Raising the pH of urine can reduce the loss of tocainide in urine.
	Cimetidine	May reduce bioavailability and serum levels. Ranitidine appears not to interact.
	Rifampicine (Rifampin)	The loss from the body may be increased by the concurrent use.

Antibiotics and Antiinfectives[1, 2]

Drugs	Interaction with	Effects
Aminoglycoside antibiotics	Amphotericin	Nephrotoxicity attributed to the concurrent use.
	Cephalosporins	Nephrotoxic effects can be increased by concurrent use which may possibly be true for other aminoglycosides.
Aminoglycosides	Clindamycin	Three cases of acute renal failure have been attributed by concurrent use.
	Dimenhydrinate	The manufactures suggest that it may considerables mask the ototoxic effects of antibiotics.
	Ethacrynic acid	Concurrent use should be avoided because of their damaging action on the ear. Intravenous administration and renal impairment are additional causative factors. Sequential use is not safe.
	Extended spectrum penicillin	Gentamicin, netilmicin, tobramicin, and sisomicin are chemically inactivated if mixed in the fluids with carbenicillin, ticarcillin, piperacillins and mezlocillin.
	Frusemide (Furosemide) or Bumetanide	May develop nephrotoxicity and/or toxicity while taking both drugs.
	Indomethacin	No authentic report on effects.
	Magnesium salts	Respiratory arrest occurred in a baby.
	Miconazole	A report describes a reduction in serum level.
	Penicillin V	The serum levels can be halved by concurrent use when given orally.
Aminoglycosides	Vancomycin	Nephrotoxicity may be additive.

Contd...

Drugs	Interaction with	Effects
Aminoglycosidic acid (PAS)	Alcohol	Can nullify the blood-lipid-lowering effects of PAS.
	Aspirin and Salicylates	Additive gastrointestinal irritation is possible. No report on other adverse effects.
	Diphenhydramine	May reduce the absorption to a little extent but clinial importance is uncertain.
	Probenecid	Serum levels may be increased by two to four folds by concurrent use.
Amphotericin	Corticosteroids	May cause potassium loss as well as salt and water retention can have adverse effect on cardiac function.
	Low salt diet	Renal toxicity and sodium depletion.
Ampicillin or Amoxycillin	Allopurinol	The incidence of skin rashes is increased by the concurrent use.
Antibiotics	Alcohol	Normally no adverse effect is reported.
Anti-infective agents	Cimetidine	No adverse effect is reported.
Anti-malarials	Antacids, antidiarrhoeals	Absorption may be reduced by 20% by the use of magnesium and about 30% by kaolin.
Cephalosporins	Cholestyramine	Absorption is delayed, importance of which is very small.
	Frusemide (Furosemide)	Nephrotoxoic effects may be increased by concurrent use of frusemide and levels in the brain are reduced as well.
Cephalosporins	Penicillins	Reduce the less from the body.
	Probenecid	Serum levels of many but not all are raised by the concurrent use.
Cephalothin	Colistin sulphomethate sodium	Renal failure is reported on concurrent use.
Chloramphenicol	Paracetamol (Acetaminophen)	May increase, decresae or to have no effect on serum levels.
	Penicillin, Streptomycin or Cephalosporins	Antagonism has been described in a case.

Contd...

Drugs	Interaction with	Effects
	Phenobarbitone	Serum levels may be depressed supported by studies in children. A single report suggests increased serum levels.
	Rifampicin	Serum levels may be markedly lowered on additional treatment.
	Cimetidine or Ranitidine	Cimetidine reduces metabolism and loss of chlorquinine from the body. Ranitidine does not interact.
Cotrimoxazole	Folic acid	The effects of folic acid may be reduced.
	Kaolin-pectin	Very small action with no clinical importance.
	Prilocaine-lignocain (Lidocain) cream	Methaemoglobinamia may develop in a body.
Cycloserine	Alcohol, Isoniazid, Phynytoin	May increase the effects of alcohol and phenytoin CNS side-effects are increased by isoniazid.
	Clofazimine	May reduce the anti-inflammatory effects.
Dapsone	Probencid	The serum levels can be raised by concurrent use.
	Rifampicin (Rifampin)	Increases the excretion of dapsone and thus lowers its serum levels.
	Antacids	May prolong the absorption time without any clinical importance.
Erythromycin	Other antibiotics	The effectiveness may be more and sometimes less effective than with only one antibiotic.
	Urinary acidifier or alkalinizers	Activity is maximal in alkaline urine and minimal in acid urine.
Ethambutol	Antacids	Aluminum hydroxide causes small reduction in the absorption with no clinical importance.
Ethinamide	Miscellaneous drugs	May cause mental depression, psychiatric disturbances, hypoglycemia, hypothyroidism and alcohol related psychotoxicity.

Contd...

Drugs	Interaction with	Effects
Flucytosine	Cytarabine	May oppose the activity.
	Miscellaneous drugs	No interaction of clinical importance.
Griseofulvin	Phenobarbitone	Anti-fungal activity may be reduced and even abolished by concurrent use.
Hexamine compounds	Urinary acidifier or alkalinizers and sulphonamides	Urinary alkalinizers and these antacids capable of raising pH above 5 should not be used. Older less soluble sulphonamides may cause the risk of kidney damage due to crystalluria as the low urinary pH values.
8-hydroxyquinoline	Zinc oxide	Inhibits the therapeutic effects in ointments.
Imipenem	Aminoglycosides	Nephrotoxic effects may be there.
Influenza vaccine	Paracetamol (Acetaminophen), Alprazolum and Lorazepam	Does not affect.
Interferon	Aspirin, Paracetamol, Prednisone	No evidence of interaction excepting that Prednisone may reduce the biological activities.
Isoniazide	Antacids	Absorption may be reduced by concurrent use. The Isoniazid may be given at least an hour. before the antacid to minimize the effects of interaction.
	Cheese or Fish	May experience a reaction with headachem, difficulty in breathing, nausea and trachycardia.
	Cimetidine or Ranitidine	No interaction reported.
	Disulfirum	Difficulties in co-ordination and changes in affects and behavior by concurrent use are reported.
	Ethambutol	Optic neuropathy may be increased by concurrent use.
	Food	Absorption is markedly reduced.
	Levodopa	Hypertension, tachycardia, flushing and tremor by concurrent use are reported.

Contd…

Drugs	Interaction with	Effects
Isoniazid	Pethidine (Meperidine)	An isolated report describes hypotension and lethargy following concurrent use.
	Propanolol	May cause reduction in the clearance from the body.
	Rifampicin	Hepatotoxicity, acetylators in presence may be increased.
Ketoconazole	Antacids and/or Cimetidine	Reduce the gastrointestinal absorption of ketoconazole.
Ketoconazole or Itraconazole	**Food**	Though the normal trends suggest the use with food, background evidence supporting this is confusing & contradictory.
	Phenytoin and phenobarbitone	Reduction in serum levels and relapse in the treatment of a fungal infection is reported.
	Rifampicin (Rifampin) and Isonizid	50-90% reduction in serum levels is reported by concurrent use.
Lincomycin or Clindamycin	**Food or drinks**	Serum levels may be depressed by up to two-thirds if taken in presence of food but clindamycin is not significantly affected.
	Kaolin	Absorption may be reduced which may be avoided by giving lincomycin 2 hr after kaolin.
Metronidazole	Antacid, kaolin-pectin and cholestyramine	Absorption is unaffected by Kaolin-pectin but small reduction occurs if aluminum hydroxide antacid is given.
	Barbiturates	Increases the loss from the body.
	Chloroquine	An isolated report describes acute dystonia.
	Cimetidine	May increase the loss to some extent with very small clinical importance.
Metronidazole	Corticosteroids	May increases the loss from the body suggesting the increased dosage of metronidazole.
	Disulfirum	Acute psychoses and confusion is reported by concurrent use.

Contd...

Drugs	Interaction with	Effects
Nalidixic acid	Nitrofurantoin	Uncertain in clinical practice.
	Probenecid	Serum levels is markedly increased by the concurrent use.
Nitrofurantoin	Antacids	Effectiveness in the treatment of urinary tract infections is reduced markedly by magnesium trisilicate, but aluminum hydroxide is reported not to interact.
	Anti-cholinergics and Diphenoxylate	May double the absorption in some patients.
Penicillins	Chloroquine	Absorption may be reduced by concurrent use but bacampicillin is not affected.
	Dietary fibre	May reduce the absorption.
	Miscellaneous drugs	Aspirin, Indomethacin, Probenecid, phenylbutazone, sulphaphenazole. Prolong the half life whereas chlorothiazide, sulphamethizole, sulphamethoxypyridazine do not.
	Tetracyclins	May reduce the effectiveness in scarlet fever.
Piperazine	Phenothiazines	Convulsion in a child was reported.
Priziquantel	Corticosteroids	Continuous use can reduce serum levels by 50%.
Primaquine (Quinacrine)	Mepacrine	Does not affect adversely.
Prothionamide	Rifampicin (Rifampin) and/or Dapson	Hypertoxicity may appear.
Pyrantel	Piperazine	May opposes the anthelmintic action.
Pyrazinamide	Miscellaneous drugs	Pyrazinamide may cause hyperuricaemia which may be modestly reduced by aminosalicylic acid or probenecid but more extensively by aspirin. May have adverse effect on control of diabetes.
	Cotrimoxazole or Sulphonamide	Pancytopemia and megaloblastic anaemia is reported.

Contd...

Drugs	Interaction with	Effects
Quinine	Antacids or Urinary acidifier and alkalinizers	Alkalinizers may increase the retension time in man but reduce in animals.
	Cimetidine or Ranitidine	Loss may be reduced by concurrent use.
	Rifampicin (Rifampin)	Serum levels may reduce.
Quinolone antibiotics	Antacids	Serum levels may reduce by concurrent use of aluminum and magnesium antacids.
	Cimetidine or Ranitidine	Cimetidine reduces the clearance from the body whereas ranitidine reduces the absorption.
	Iron preparations	May reduce the absorption of ciprofloxacin and ofloxacin. Quinolone-iron complexes formed have reduced antibacterial effects.
	Rifampicin (Rifampin)	Serum levels may be reduced but no interaction was reported.
Quinolone antibiotics	Sucralfate	Causes marked reduction in the absorption if taken together but a smaller reduction is reported if dosage are separated by 2hr.
	Zinc	May reduce absorption.
Rifampicin	Aminosalicylic acid (PAS)	Serum levels may be halved.
Rifampicin (Rifampin)	Antacids	Reduction up to 30% may be caused by concurrent use with uncertain clinical importance.
	Clofazimine	No interaction is reported.
	Dipyrone	No significant interaction.
	Food	May delays and reduce the absorption.
	Probenecid	Unpredictable.
	Triacetyloleandomycin	Cholestatic jaundice have been reported.
Rifampentine	Other drugs	Have ten times greater potency and a linger half-life. So far no clinical important interaction reported.

Contd...

Drugs	Interaction with	Effects
Sulphasalazine	Antibiotics	The release in the colon of the active drug is markedly reduced by concurrent use.
Sulphasalazine or Sodium fusidate	Cholestyramine	Cholestyramine can bind with two drugs thereby reducing their activity.
Sulphasalazine	Iron salts	May bind but the therapeutic response is uncertain.
Suphasalazine	Metronidazole	Does not interact.
	Barbiturates	Anaestetic effects are increased but shortened.
	Local anaesthetics	May reduce the effects and allow the development of local and generalized infections.
	Para-aminobenzoic acid (PABA)	Antibacterial effects are reduced.
Tetracyclins	Alcohol	Serum levels may fall below minimal therapeutic concentration but tetracyclin itself is not affected.
	Antacids	Effectiveness may be reduced markedly and even abolished by concurrent use of antacids containing aluminum, bismuth, calcium or magnesium. Other antacids may raise the gastric pH.
	Anticonvulsants	The serum levels may be reduced and may fall below the accepted therapeutic minimum.
	Cimetidine	Does not interact.
	Colestipol	May markedly reduce the absorption.
	Diuretics	Concurrent use should be avoided because of their association with rises in blood urea nitrogen level.
	Iron preparations	Absorption from the gut of both is remarkably reduced by concurrent use which leads to depressed serum levels.

Contd...

Drugs	Interaction with	Effects
		Effectiveness may be reduced and even abolished.
	Milk and diary products	Absorption may be remarkably reduced if comes in contact in gut leading to reduction and even abolishment of therapeutic effects. Doxycyclin is the least affected.
	Rifampicin (Rifampin)	Serum levels may be reduced up to 50%.
Tetracyclins	Thiomarsal	May experience on inflammatory ocular reaction.
	Zinc sulphate	Reduction as much as 50% is reported.
Tinidazole	Rifampicin (Rifampin)	Increases the loss from the body.
Trimethoprine	Antacids	Magnesium trisilicate and kaolin-pectin reduce the bioavailability of trimethoprine with uncertain clinical importance.
	Guar or food	May reduce the absorption.
Vidarabine	Allopurinol	Toxicity of vidarabine may be increased by concurrent use.
Zidovudine (Azidothymidine)	Miscellaneous drugs	Paracetamol increases the haematological toxicity to considerable extent but acyclovir, aspirin, ketoconazole, and cotrimoxazole appear not to interact.

Anticoagulants[1, 2]

Drugs	Interaction with	Effects
	ACE inhibitors	No interaction reported.
	Acitretin	Does not alter the effects.
Anticoagulants	Alcohol	No alteration of effects who drinks small or moderate amount of alcohol but clronic alcoholic with liver disease shows fluctuation in prothrombin times.

Contd...

Drugs	Interaction with	Effects
	Allopurinol	No adverse interaction on oral administration in most patients but monitoring the initial anticoagulant response is necessary since excessive hypoprothrombinaemia and bleeding may occur.
	Aminoglutethinide	Concurrent use may reduce the effectiveness remarkably.
	Aminoglycoside antibiotics	If the intake of vitamin K is normal, either small or no interaction takes place.
	Aminosalicylic acid (PAS) and/or Isomiazid	A report describes anticoagulant response on concurrent use.
	Amiodarone	Effectiveness may be increased and bleeding may occur if dosage is not being reduced.
	Anabolic steroids and related sex hormones	Anticoagulant effects are markedly increased by concurrent use. Bleeding may occur if dosage is not changed/reduced appropriately.
	Antacids	Aluminum hydroxide does not interact with warfarin or dicoumarol and magnesium hydroxide does not interact with warfarin. Evidence supports that absorption may be increased by magnesium hydroxide with no clinical supports.
	Ascorbic acid (Vitamin C)	Isolated case describes that effectiveness may be reduced.
	Aspirin and other salicylates	Aspirin in doses of 500 mg/day increases the bleeding 3-5 times.
	Azapropazone	The effectiveness may be increased and bleeding may occur if dosage is not reduced.
	Barbiturates	The effectiveness may be reduced. 30-60% increase in dosage is required to obtain full therapeutic effects.
	Benfluorex	Does not alter the effects.

Contd...

Drugs	Interaction with	Effects
	Benziodarone	The effectiveness is increased. The dosage should be reduced approximately.
	Benzodiazepines	The anticoagulant effects are not affected.
	Benzydamine hydrochloride	The effects are not altered.
	Beta-blockers	Oral anticoagulants are not affected by the concurrent use.
	5-bromo-2-deoxyuridine (BUDR)	The effectiveness is markedly increased.
	Calcium channel blockers	Does not interact adversely.
	Carbamazepine	The effectiveness may be markedly reduced. The dosage needs to be doubled.
	Carbon tetrachloride	Single report describes the increment in the effectiveness
	Cephalosporins	May increase the effectiveness.
	Chloral hydrate	The effectiveness may be increased but this is of little or no clinical importance.
	Chloramphenicol	Concurrent use may increase the effectiveness.
	Cholestyramine or Colestipol	The effectiveness may be reduced.
	Cimetidine, Ranitidine or Nizatidine	The effectiveness may be increased by concurrent use of cimetidine. Ranitidine and nizatidine does not interact.
	Cinclophen	Concurrent use may increase the effectiveness. Bleeding occurs if the dosage is not reduced appropriately.
	Cisapride	May cause a small increase in the effectiveness.
	Clofibrate, Bezafibrate or Gemfibrozil	Bleeding may occur with the increment in the effectiveness so dosage should be reduced appropriately.

Contd...

Drugs	Interaction with	Effects
Anticoagulants	Contraceptives (oral) and Sex Related hormones	The effects of dicoumarol can be increased but for nicoumalone, the effect may be decreased by the concurrent use.
	Corticosteroids or ACTH	Unpredictable but small change may occur.
	Cytotoxic (antineoplastic) agents	Concurrent use may increase the effectiveness supported by single report. A decrease in the effects is also reported with cyclophosphamide, reaptopurine and mitotane.
	Dextropropoxyphene	Five patients showed a marked increase in the effects.
	Dichloralphenazone	The effectiveness is reduced by the concurrent use.
	Diflunisal	Limited causes describes the increment of the effects with warfarin but phenprocoumon appear not to interact.
	Dipyridamol	Mild bleeding may occur on concurrent use.
	Dipyrone	One report describes no interaction while another claims a rapid but transient increase in the effectiveness.
	Disopyramide	Effectiveness may be reduced but reverse report is also there.
	Disulfiram	May increase the effectiveness. Bleeding may occur if dosage is not reduced appropriately.
	Ditazole	No alteration of effects reported.
	Diuretics	Does not affect the effectiveness. Rare occurrence in the increase in the effects is reported with ethacrynic acid. Bleeding may occur.
	Erythromycin	Increase in the effects associated with bleeding is reported.
	Ethchlorvynol	Effectiveness may be well reduced by concurrent use.

Contd...

Drugs	Interaction with	Effects
	Fenofibrate (procetofene)	Increase in the effectiveness with bleeding is reported unless the anticoagulant dose is reduced by one-third.
	Feprazone	Effectiveness may be increased.
	Flutamide	May increase the effects.
	Food	Rate of absorption is increased. Soy protein may reduce the absorption rate.
	Glucagon	Effectiveness is rapidly and markedly increased in large doses. Bleeding may occur if warfarin dosage is not reduced appropriately.
	Glutethimide	Concurrent use may reduce the effects.
	Griseofulvin	Effectiveness may be reduced by concurrent use.
	Halofenate	Increase in the effects by concurrent use is reported.
	Haloperidol	Concurrent use may reduce the effectiveness.
	Heparinoid	Bleeding is reported by a single report.
	Herbal remedies	Herbal remedies itself containing anticoagulating effects is expected to increase the effectiveness.
Anticoagulants	Hydrocodone	Effects may be increased.
	Indomethacin	No particular case is reported to have altered effectiveness. Caution is required to be taken because indomethacin may cause irritation and bleeding.
	Influenza vaccines	Concurrent use is safe but report of bleeding is attributed to an interaction.
	Insecticides	An isolated report describes a patient having forted to respond after very heavy exposure to an insecticide.

Contd...

Drugs	Interaction with	Effects
	Isoxicam and Peroxicam	Effectiveness may be increased.
	Ketoconazole	Three elderly patients showed increase in the effects. But no interaction is also reported.
	Laxatives, Liquid Paraffin or Psyllium	No change either in the absorption rate or anticoagulant effects is reported.
	Meclofenamic acid or Mefenamic acid	Increase in the effectiveness is reported.
	Meprobamate	After the effectiveness in significant amounts.
	Meptazinol	No change in the effects is reported.
	Methaqualone	May cause small change but clinically unimportant.
	Methylphenidate	No change in the effects is reported.
	Methonidazole	May cause marked increase in the effects. Bleeding may occur if dosage is not altered appropriately.
	Miconazole	Effectiveness may be markedly increased on concurrent use. Bleeding may occur if dosage is not reduced appropriately.
	Monoamine oxidase inhibitors	No confirmed clinical report is attributed.
	Nalidixic acid	Two out of three developed hyporpothrombinaemia and one reported bleeding.
	Nizatidine	Does not interact.
	Nomifensine	A single report supports the increase in effectiveness.
	Non-steroidal antiinflammatory drugs (NSAID's) Arylalkanoates	Effectiveness may be increased in few patients and may bleed. No interaction takes place with normal doses.
	Omeprazole	May cause very small change in the effectiveness.

Contd...

Drugs	Interaction with	Effects
	Oxametacin	Concurrent use may increase the effects.
Anticoagulants	Oxpentifylline	No significant change in effects by concurrent use.
	Paracetamol (Acetaminophen)	No significant change in the effects is reported.
	Penicillins	No change takes place on oral administration of anticoagulants but isolated report describes increased prothrombin times and bleeding also occur. Isolated case also supports the reduction in the effectiveness.
	Phenazone (Antipyrine)	Effectiveness may be reduced.
	Phenothiazines	Does not interact.
	Phenylbutazone	Effectiveness is markedly increased by concurrent use. To avoid bleeding, concurrent use may be restricted.
	Phenyramidol	Increase in effects associated with bleeding may takes place. So, reduction in dosage is recommended.
	Piracetam	A single report describes who began to bleed within a month of starting to take piracetam.
	Prolintane	No alteration in the effectiveness is reported.
	Profagenone	Concurrent use may cause increase in the effectiveness. Reduction in the dosage is necessary.
	Proquatone	No change in the effects.
	Quinidine	Effectiveness may be increased with bleeding. A decrease in the effect is also reported.
	Quinine	No change in the effects is reported on oral administration.

Contd...

Drugs	Interaction with	Effects
	Quinolone antibiotics	Enoxacin does not interact, nor ciprofloxacin with nicoumalane or ethylbicoumacelate nor ofloxacin with phenprocoumon. Increase in the effect is also reported.
	Rifampicin (Rifampin)	Concurrent use may reduce the effectiveness which demands the dosage to be increased accordingly.
	Reoprostil	May reduce the effectivenees.
	Roxithromycin	Does not interact.
	Simvastatin	May cause small but clinically unimportant increase in the effectiveness.
	Sucralfate	Two cases describe marked reduction in the effects. Uncommon interaction is also reported.
	Sulindac	Occasional increase in the effectiveness is reported.
	Suloctidil or Zomepirac	Does not intertact significantly.
	Sulphinpyrazone	May increase the effects markedly associated with serious bleeding provided the dosage is not reduced appropriately.
	Sulphonamides	Concurrent use may increase the effects. Bleeding may occur if dosage is not changed appropriately.
	Tomaxifen	Concurrent use may increase the effects significantly. Reduction in dosage by a half and even more may be necessary to avoid bleeding.
	Terodiline	Does not alter the effects.
	Tetracycline, Tricylic and other antidepressants	Oral anticoagulants donot alter the effects. A single report describes increase in the effectiveness with mianserin and lofepramine.

Contd...

Drugs	Interaction with	Effects
	Tetracycline	Generally no change in the effects is reported. Isolated case describes increase in the effects.
	Thyroid or Antithyroid compounds	Concurrent use may increase the effects. Bleeding may occur if dosage is not reduced appropriately. A reduction in the effectiveness is expected if antithyroid compounds are used.
	Ticlopidine	The concurrent use may cause liver damage.
	Trazodone	Concurrent use can be uneventful while an isolated case describes a woman who needed increased dosage.
	Vitamin E	Limited cases are reported that it may increase or decrease effectiveness.
	Vitamin K	Effectiveness may be reduced and even abolished by the concurrent use.
Heparin	Aspirin	May be effective in the prevention of post-operative thromboembolism but risk of bleeding occur.
	Dextran	Although successful and uneventful evidence is also there which suggests the increment of the effectiveness. Dosage may be reduced to a third or a half during concurrent use.
	Glyceryl trinitrate (Nitroglycerin)	The effectiveness may be reduced by concurrent use.
	Probenecid	May possibly increase the effectiveness associated with bleeding.

Anticonvulsants Drugs[1,2]

Drugs	Interaction with	Effects
Anticonvulsants	Acetazolamide	Severe osteomalacia and rickets is reported by concurrent use. A marked reduction in serum level is also attributed.
	Aspartame	May cause convulsions.
	Calcium channel blockers	Verapamil may cause marked rise in serum level which is also similar with dilitiazem. Nifedipine does not interact, but may cause phenytoin intoxication. The serum level of felodipine may markedly deduced by carbamazepine, phenobarbitone and phenytoin.
	Cinromide	May depress the serum level.
	Cytotoxic drugs	Serum level may be reduced markedly by concurrent use with cytotoxic drugs.
	Denzimol	Marked and rapid rise in serum level accompanied by acute toxicity is reported.
	Dextropropryphene	Concurrent use may rise the serum level associated with toxicity.
	Disulfiram	Serum levels are markedly and rapidly increased by concurrent use.
	Felbamate	May raise the serum level.
	Folic acid	Fall in the serum levels leading to adverse seizure control may occur by concurrent use.
	Influenza vaccines	May rise in the serum level.
	Nafimidone	May raise the serum level. Dosage reduction is needed to prevent toxicity.
	Progabide	Serum level can rise by concurrent use.
	Pyridoxine	Large dose (200mg daily) can cause reduction up to 40-50% in the serum level.

Contd...

Drugs	Interaction with	Effects
	Quinolone antibiotics	Ciprofloxacin and enoxacin may cause occational convulsions.
	Stiriprentol	May cause marked rise in serum levels, Dosage to be reduced to avoid toxicity.
	Tobacco smoking	No important interaction.
	Vigabatrin	May reduce in serum level.
	Viloxazine	Serum levels may rise up to 50% by concurrent use.
Barbiturates	Caffeine	The hypnotic effects may be reduced and even abolished by concurrent use.
	Cimetidine	May reduce the absorption of cimetidine.
	Miconazole	Serum levels may be increased.
	Rifampicin (Rifampin)	May markedly increase the clearance from the body. The effects of both are expected to be reduced.
	Sodium valproate	Concurrent use may cause the increase in serum levels. A reduction in the dosage by a third to a half can be safely carried out.
	Triacetylobandomycin	Concurrent use may cause marked reduction in the serum levels.
Carbamazepine or Phenobarbitone	Benzodiazepines	No effects reported but serum level may be reduced of limited clinical importance.
	Cimetidine or Ranitidine	Transient increase in serum levels is reported. Cimetidine appears to produce some side effect, which disappears rapidly. Ranitidine does not interact.
	Danazol	Concurrent use may rise in the serum level. Dosage reduction in recommended to avoid toxicity.
	Diuretics	Hyponatraemia may be caused by concurrent use.

Contd...

Drugs	Interaction with	Effects
Carbamazepine	Erythromycin	Serum levels may be raised rapidly to toxic concentration by concurrent use. Erythromycin does not interact with Phenytoin.
	Isoniazid	Concurrent use may rise the serum level rapidly. Reduced dosage is required to avoid intoxication.
	Macrolide antibiotics	Serum level may rise rapidly leading to intoxication within 1-3 days.
	Miconazole	A single report describes adverse response by concurrent use.
	Monoamine oxidase inhibition	No interaction is reported.
	Phenobarbitone	Reduction in serum levels is reported by concurrent use.
	Primidone	Marked reduction in serum levels is reported.
	Sodium valproate	Serum levels of both may fall by 20-25% by concurrent use.
	Valpromide	Intoxication (carbamazepine) may occur if valpromide is not replaced by sodium valproate.
Ethosuximide	Barbiturates, Phenytoin or Primidone	Fall in the serum levels may be caused by concurrent use. Phenytoin intoxication is also reported.
	Carbamazepine	Serum levels may be reduced.
	Isoniazid	An isolated report describes psychotic behaviour and signs of ethosuximide intoxication by concurrent use.
	Sodium valproate	Significant rise in the serum levels is reported by concurrent use.
Phenytoin	Alcohol	Chronic heavy drinking reduces serum concentration. Excessive drinking also increases the frequency of seizures in epileptics.
	Allopurinol	A single report describes intoxication in a body by concurrent use.

Contd...

Drugs	Interaction with	Effects
	Amiodarone	Serum levels may be raised. Phenytoin intoxication may occur if dosage is not reduced appropriately.
	Antacids	Some, but not all cases can reduce serum level.
	Anticoagulants	Serum level may be increased. Effectiveness may be reduced.
	Aspirin	Phenytoin toxicity is reported. Adverse interaction occurs in most patients.
	Azapropazone	Concurrent use may rise in the serum levels. Phenytoin intoxication is likely to develop.
	Barbiturates	Concurrent use is uneventful. Phenytoin intoxication has been reported.
	Benzodiazepines	May cause to rise, fall or remain unaltered in the serum levels.
	Carbamazepine	Rise or fall in the serum levels are reported by concurrent use.
	Chloramphenicol	Concurrent use may rise the serum levels. Phenytoin intoxication in two patients.
	Chlorpheniramine	Concurrent use reports phenytoin intoxication in two patients.
	Cholestyramine or Colestipol	No change in absorption rate is reported.
	Cimetidine, Famotidine and Ranitidine	Serum levels may be raised by cimetidine with toxicity. Others two donot react with phenytoin.
	Cloxacillin	Concurrent use may cause marked reduction in serum levels.
	Diazoxide	Reports of four children who showed marked reduction in serum levels are attributed with reduced effectiveness.
	Dichloralphenazone	Concurrent use may lead to reduction in serum levels.

Contd...

Drugs	Interaction with	Effects
	Floconazole	Serum levels may rise rapidly. Toxicity may develop if dosage is not being reduced appropriately.
	Food	The absorption may be affected by some food.
	Carbapentin	Concurrent use shows no interaction of clinical importance.
	Hypoglycaemic agents	Large and toxic doses may cause hyperglycaemia.
	Ibuprofen	No interaction of clinical importance is reported.
	Influenza vaccines	Reports to increase decrease or to have no effects on the serum levels have been documented.
	Isoniazid	Serum levels may be raised by concurrent use.
	Loxapine	Depressed serum levels by concurrent use is reported.
	Methylphenidate	Serum levels may be raised associated with intoxication.
	Metronidazole	Small and clinically unimportant rise in the serum level is reported.
	Miconazole	Intoxication is reported in two cases.
	Omeprazole	The loss from the body is reduced.
	Pheneturide	Serum levels may be raised up to 50% by concurrent use.
	Phenothiazines	Serum levels may be raised or lowered.
	Phenylbutazone	Serum levels may be raised. Intoxication may appear if dosage is not reduced appropriately.
	Phenyramidol	Serum levels may be raised upto three folds by concurrent use. Phenytoin dosage is to be reduced to avoid intoxication.
	Rifampicin (Rifampin)	Clearance is doubled by the concurrent use.
	Sodium valproate	Uneventful.

Contd...

Drugs	Interaction with	Effects
	Sucralfate	The absorption may be reduced to 7-20% by concurrent use.
	Suiphinpyrazone	Concurrent use may rise the serum levels markedly. Dosage is to be reduced appropriately to avoid intoxication.
	Sulphonamides	Serum levels may be raised by co-trimoxazole, suiphamethizole, suiphamethoxazole, trimethoprinete by concurrent use. Others like sulphadimethoxine etc. don't interact.
	Sulthiame	Concurrent use may raise the serum levels to double resulting intoxication if dosage is not being reduced appropriately.
	Theophyllin	Serum levels and effectiveness may be markedly reduced by concurrent use leading to need of increment in dosage to maintain concentration.
	Teinilic acid (Ticrynoden)	Intoxication is reported.
	Trazodone	Concurrent use may result intoxication.
	Tricyclic antidepressants	Very limited evidence supports that serum level may be raised by concurrent use.
Primidone	Barbiturates	Elevated serum phenobarbitone levels may develop by concurrent use.
	Carbamazepine, Clonazepam or Clorazepate	Carbamazepine may reduce but clonazepam may raise the serum level.
	Isoniazid	Serum level may be reduced by concurrent use.
	Phenytoin	Concurrent use may raise the serum level.
	Sodium valproate	Serum levels may be increased or decreased by concurrent use.

Contd...

Drugs	Interaction with	Effects
Sodium valproate	Antacids	Absorption is slightly accelerated by (aluminium-magnesium hydroxide) but no interaction with magnesium trisilicate or calcium carbonate.
	Aspirin	Large dose may develop toxicity by concurrent use. Blood levels increased by aspirin.
	Benzodiazepines	Side effects may be increased.
	Cimetidine or Ranitidine	Cimetidine interacts minimally whereas ranitidine does not.
	CNS depressants and alcohol	Potentiate the activity of Sodium Valproate.

Antihypertensives[1,2]

Drugs	Interaction with	Effects
ACE inhibitors	Allopurinol	Concurrent use may cause serious Stevens-Johnson syndrome and hypersensitivity.
	Antacids	May reduce the absorption by concurrent use.
	Azathiprine	Leucopenia in the occational case may be resulted by concurrent use.
	Diuretic	Generally safe and effective. But a few patients may have felt lightheaded within an hour of first dose resulting hypotension. Hyperkalaemia is also possible if potassium-sparing or potassium supplements are used.
	Non-steroidal antiinflammatory drugs	The effectiveness may be reduced or even abolished by imdomethacin, ibuprofen and aspirin.
	Other antihypertensives	The effects may be delayed to occur. Dosage reduction is required to avoid hypotension.
Acetazolamide	Beta-blockers	Patients with chronic obstructive lung disease may witness acidosis.

Contd...

Drugs	Interaction with	Effects
Amlodipine + Linisopril	Diuretics	Fall in BP, hypocalaemia with concommitant use of potassium sparing diuretics.
	Indomethacin	It may alternate antihypertensive effect of linisopril.
	Thiazides	Linisopril reduce the potassium loss.
Antihypertensives	Alcohol	Blood pressure may be raised by moderate to heavy drinking. Postural hypertensive, dizziness and fainting shortly after having a drink may also be experienced.
	Fenfluramine	May increase the blood pressure thus lowering the effectiveness.
	Food	Absorption may remain unaltered and if lowers, very little.
	Phenothiazine	Side effects of phenothizines may increase the side effects of others, the patients may fell faint if they stand up quickly.
	Pyrazolone compounds	Effectiveness may be reduced.
	Salbutamol	Severe hypotension is reported.
Atenolol	Indomethacin	Reduces antihypertensive effect of atenolol.
Benazepril	Diuretics	Increases the risk of hyperkalaemia.
	Thiazides	Excessive fall in blood pressure.
	Food	Rate of absorption delayed.
Bisoprolol	Anaesthetic agents, clonidine, calcium antagonists, digitalis, hypoglycaemic agents, NSAIDs.	The action of these Drugs are enhanced by Bisoprolol.
	Rifampicin	May cause reduction in plasma concentration and elimination half-life of the Bisoprolol.
Captopril	Immunosuppressive Drugs	Risk of bone marrow depression increased.
	Probenecids	It delays the excretion of captopril and increases the blood level of captopril.
	Morphine	The analgesic and respiratory depression produced by morphine may be accentuated by captopril.

Contd...

Drugs	Interaction with	Effects
Carvedilol	Rifampicin	Pretreatment with rifampicin results in a decreased C_{max} and AUC.
	Verapamil	Severe bradycardia and myocardial depression.
	Clonidine	Hypotensive and cardiodepressive actions are potentiated.
Clonidine	Beta-blockers	Concurrent use may cause a sharp and serious rise in blood pressure. The effectiveness may also be abolished which is reported.
Clonidine or Apomorphine	Oral contraceptives	Concurrent use may reduce the sedative effects.
Clonidine	Prazosin	Effectiveness may be reduced by concurrent use.
	Tricyclic antidepressants	Reduction or even abolition of effectiveness may be reduced.
Diazoxide	Hypoglycaemic agents and hypotensive agents	Severe hypotension is reported. Excessive hypoglycaemia may also occur by concurrent use.
Diltiazem	Digoxin, Cyclosporine	Elevates serum digoxin and cyclosporin levels.
	Propanolol	Potentiate the action of propanolol.
	Cimetidine	It may increase the plasma concentration of diltiazem.
Diuretics (Potassium-sparing)	Potassium suppliments and salt subastitutes	Severe and life threatening hyperkalaemia may result if potassium level is not monitored.
Diuretics	Trimethoprium	Excessive low serum levels are reported by concurrent use.
Enalapril	Cyclophosphamide, Azathioprine	Risk of bone marrow suppression increased with concomitant therapy with the immunosuppressive Drugs.
Enalapril	Diuretics/Potassium Supplements	Hyperkalaemia and potentiates the hypotensive action.
	Probenecids	It delays the excretion of the enalapril.
	Morphine	Potentiates the analgesia and respiratory depression produced by morphine.

Contd...

Drugs	Interaction with	Effects
Frusemide	Chloralhydrate	Intravenous injection of frusemide after being treated with chloral may cause sweating, hot flushes, a variable blood pressure.
	Clofibrate	Diuresis and muscular symptoms are reported by concurrent use.
	Food	May reduce the bioavailability of frusemide and diuretic effects.
Frusemide or Bumetanide	Indomethacins and others NSAID's	The antihypertension and diuretic effects may be reduced or even abolished by concurrent use.
	Phenytoin	The effectiveness may be reduced up to 50% by the concurrent use.
	Probenacid	May cause the reduction of urinary loss of sodium.
Guanethidine and related drugs	Haloperidol or Thiothixene	Concurrent use may reduce the effectiveness.
	Indirectly acting sympathomimetic amines and related drugs	Concurrent use reduces the effectiveness to even abolition. Blood pressure may be increased.
	Monoamine oxidase inhibitors	The effects may be reduced by the concurrent use.
	Phenothiazines	Large doses may cause reduction or even abolition of the effectiveness by the concurrent use.
	Pizotifen	The effectiveness may be even abolished.
	Tricyclic antidepressants	The effects may be reduced and even abolished by the concurrent use.
	Tyramine – rich foods	Serious hypertension is reported.
Hydralazine	Diclofenac	Diclofenac is reported to oppose the effectiveness of hydralazine. It is uncertain in the case of indomethacin.
Indapamide	Thiazide/Potassium losing diuretics	Hypokalaemia and hypercalcuria enhanced.
Indoramin	Alcohol	Concurrent use may raise the serum levels of both.

Contd...

Drugs	Interaction with	Effects
Ketanserin	Beta-blockers	Acute hypotension has been reported by the concurrent use.
	Diuretics	Sudden deaths, abnormal heart rhythm may be markedly increased by concurrent use.
Labetalol	Halothane	Hypotensive effect of halothane enhanced by labetalol.
	Anti-arrythmics & antagonists	Potentiates action of anti-arrythmics and Ca-antagonists.
	Cimetidine	Bio-availability of labetalol increases.
Lacidipine	Cimetidine	It increases the plasma lacidipine levels.
Linisopril	Indomethacin	It may reduce the hypotensive effect of linisopril.
	Hydrochlorthiazide	Hypotensive effect of linisopril is potentiated leading to severe hypotension and hyperkalaemia.
Linisopril	Alcohol	Hypotensive effect of Linisopril is potentiated by alcohol.
	Cyclo-oxygenase inhibitors	Co-administration of cyclo-oxygenase inhibitors may cause sharp reduction in renal function.
	Diuretics	Hypotensive effect of Losartan is potentiated by diuretics.
Losartan potassium	NSAIDs	It may blunt anti-hypertensive response of losartan.
	Cimetidine	It may increase the AUC of Losartan by about 18%.
	Phenobarbital	It may reduce the AUC of Losartan and its active metabolite.
	Ketoconazol	It inhibits the conversion of Losartan to its active metabolites.
	Barbiturates	Concurrent use doesnot alter the effects.
Methyldopa	Cephalosporin	Pustular eruptions may occur by concurrent use.
	Disulphiram	Abolition of effectiveness may be caused.
	General anaesthetics	It enhances the effect of methyldopa.
	Haloperidol	Concurrent use may result dementia but no serious problem is reported.

Contd...

Drugs	Interaction with	Effects
	Iron salts	Concurrent use may reduce the effectiveness.
	Phenoxybenzamine	Total urinary incontinence is reported by concurrent use.
Metoprolol	Tricyclic antidepressants	Concurrent use does not adversely alter the effects but hypertension, tachycardia, tumor are reported.
	Verapamil	Hypotension, bradycardia and asystole with verapamil in the presence of AV nodal block and LVF.
	Antidiabetics	Masking of hypoglycaemic symptoms.
	Cimetidine	Metoprolol activity is potentiated.
	Nifedipine, nitrates, verapamil	Enhancement of anti-anginal activity.
	Diuretics and vasodialators	Enhancement of anti-hypertensive activity.
Nifedipine	Quinidine	Plasma quinidine levels may be reduced.
	Theophylline, phenytoin	Levels of plasma theophylline and phenytoin levels increased.
	Beta-blockers	Synergism and reduce depression of cardiac function.
	Cimetidine	Bio-availability of Nifedipine increases and hypotensive action is potentiated.
Nitrendipine	Theophylline, phenytoin	Levels of plasma theophylline and phenytoin levels increased.
	Beta-blockers	Synergism and reduce depression of cardiac function.
	Cimetidine	Bio-availability of Nitrendipine increases and hypotensive action is potentiated.
Perindopril	Diuretics	Diuretics that lead to salt depletion increase risk of hypotension with the drug, potassium sparing diuretics can cause hypokalaemia, increase in lithium level.
	NSAIDs	Reduction in anti-hypertensive effect.
Prazosin	Beta-blockers	May cause some patients to faint.

Contd…

Drugs	Interaction with	Effects
Prazosin	Calcium channel blockers	Blood pressure may fall sharply. Close monitoring of the response is required.
	Diuretics	Diuretics aggravate sodium depletion.
Propranolol	Adrenaline	Marked hypertension and bradycardia.
	Anaesthetic agents	Reduced heart rate and output.
	Digitalis & Calcium channel blockers	Severe bradycardia may occur (especially with impaired left ventricular function)
	Chlorpromazine	Blood levels of both the drug increases and additive hypotensive effect.
	Cimetidine	Blood levels of propranolol increases.
	Indomethacin	Hypotensive effect is reduced.
	Smoking	Reduced efficacy.
	Vasodilators	Trachycardia inhibited.
	Other antihypertensives and diuretics	Additive effect.
Ramipril	Diuretics	Concommitant administration may lead to serious hypotension and with potassium sparing diuretics dangerous hyperkalaemia may result. Serum lithium concentration may increase.
	NSAIDs	Effect of the drug may be reduced, and cause deterioration of renal function.
	Alcohol	Effect is exacerbated.
	Vasodilators	Inhibits trachycardia.
Rauwolfia alkaloids	Tricyclic antidepressants	May be successfully used in some resistant form of depression by concurrent use.
Sotalol	General anaesthetics	May impair myocardial contractility.
	Antidepressants & Quinidine	Polymorphic ventricular trachycardia.
Spironolactone	Dextropropoxyphene	Gynaecomastia and rash is reported.

Contd...

Drugs	Interaction with	Effects
Terazocin	Beta-blockers, calcium channel blockers, diuretics	Orthostatic hypotension is potentiated.
Thiazides	Calcium carbonate	Hypercalaemia and metabolic alkalosis is reported by concurrent use.
	Cholestyramine or Colestipol	The absorption may be reduced by the concurrent use. The diuretic effect is likely to be reduced accordingly.
	Indomethacin and other NSAID's	Reduction in the effectiveness by indomethacin of moderate clinical importance is reported. Ibuprofen has less impacts where as others interact resulting no adverse effects.
	Propantheline	May increase the absorption by concurrent use.
Triamterene	Cimetidine or Ranitidine	Ranitidine may reduce the absorption and diuretic effects of uncertain clinical importance. Cimetidine does not interact.
	Indomethacin	Acute renal failure is reported by concurrent use.

Antiparkinsonian Drugs [1, 2]

Drugs	Interaction with	Effects
Amantadine	Miscellaneous drugs	Various problems are reported.
	Thiazides	Successful and unsuccessful concurrent uses are reported. Intoxication is also reported.
Anticholinergics	Betel nuts	Controls of side effects are reported by concurrent use.
Benzohexol	Tricyclic antidepressants, antiparkinsonian Drugs, antihistaminic and quinidines	Additive anticholinergic activity.

Contd...

Drugs	Interaction with	Effects
Bromocriptine	Alcohol	Alcohol reduces tolerance to the drug and vice-versa.
	Erythromycin	Bioavailability of the bromocriptin is increased.
	Griseofulvin	Effectiveness may be opposed.
	Macrolid antibiotics	Toxicity may occur with Josamycin. Marked serum level is reported with erythromycin.
Levodopa	Anticholinergics	Effectiveness may be reduced.
	Benzodiazepines	Concurrent use may reduce and even abolish the effects.
	Beta-blockers	Concurrent use may appear favorable but long time effects of the elevated growth hormones are uncertain.
	Clonidene	The effects may be opposed by the concurrent use.
	Ferrus sulphate	May reduce the bioavailability.
	Food	May reduce the effectiveness by concurrent use.
	Methionine	Concurrent use may reduce the effects.
	Methyldopa	May cause in the increment of effects there by reduction in dose is essential.
	Metoclopramide	Some of the effects may be increased and a few may be opposed.
Levodopa	Monoamine oxidase inhibitors (MAOI)	Concurrent use may cause a rapid, serious and potentially life-threatening hypertension.

Contd…

Drugs	Interaction with	Effects
	Papaverine	May cause deterioration in the control of parkinsonism with no confirm trial report.
	Phenothiazines or Butyrophenones	Concurrent use may oppose the effects by each other.
	Phenylbutazone	The effects may be antagonised by concurrent use.
	Phenytoin	Concurrent use may reduce and even abolish the effects.
	Piperidine	Concurrent use may oppose the effectiveness.
	Pyridoxine (Vit - B6)	The effectiveness may be reduced and even abolished by the concurrent use.
	Rauwolfia alkaloids	The effects may be opposed by the concurrent use.
		The concurrent use is uneventful although very small reduction in the effectiveness is reported. Hypertensive crisis is also reported.
Orphenadrine	Anticholinergics, alcohol, other CNS depressants, MAOls and antidepressants	These drugs are potentiated by orphenadrine.
	Propoxyphene	May cause tremors and mental confusion.
	Chlorpromazine	Plasma chlorpromazine level decreased.
	Levodopa	Synergistic effects.
Selegiline	Reserpine, Tetrabenazine	Interfere with the effect of Selegiline.

Beta – blockers[1,2]

Drugs	Interaction with	Effects
Beta – blockers	Antacids	A few antacids may cause small reduction in the absorption of proporanolol, atenolol, and others while absorption may be increased with metaprolol are reported by concurrent use.
	Anticholinesterases	Bradycardia and hypotension is reported by the concurrent use.
	Barbiturates	May cause reduction in the removal process from the body by liver.
	Calcium channel blockers	Concurrent use is reported to be useful. However some level may be raised of clinical unimportance.
	Cholestyramine or Colestipol	Serum level may be reduced.
	Cimetidine	The blood levels may be doubled by the concurrent use. Bradycardia (heart rate 36 beats/min) and hypotension is also reported.
	Cimetidine phenylephrine	Lowering of blood pressure by the concurrent use is reported. Bronchospasm may also occur.
	Contraceptives (Oral)	The blood levels may be increased with uncertain clinical importance.
	Dextromoramide	Bradycardia and severe hypotension is reported.
	Diltiazem	Although mainly safe and uneventful but bradycardia is also reported.
	Ergotamine or Methylsergids	Although mainly very effective and useful but severe peripheral vasoconstriction is also described.
	Erythromycin or Neomycin	Serum levels may be increased.
	Etintidine	Serum levels may be increased.
	Food	Food may increase, decrease or have no effect on the bioavailability.
	Halofenate	Concurrent use may reduce the serum levels and the therapeutic effects.

Contd…

Drugs	Interaction with	Effects
	Haloperidol	Hypotension and cardiopulmonary assets in women may be occurred.
	Hydralozine	Serum levels may be increased with no adverse impact.
	Indomethacin and other NSAID's	Effectiveness may be reduced. Sulindac donot interact. Aspirin appears to be uncertain. Indomethacin may cause hypertension.
	Morphine	Serum levels may be increased.
	Nifedipine	Concurrent use is effective but excessive hypotension and heart failure is also reported.
	Phenothiazines	Serum levels may be increased the both. Excessive hypotension is reported.
	Propafenone	Serum levels may be raised by 2-5 folds by the concurrent use.
	Rifampicin (Rifampin)	May increase the serum levels.
	Suiphinpyrazone	Concurrent use may reduce and even abolish the effectiveness.
	Thallium scans	May provide false information of stress thallium scans, used for the diagnosis of coronary heart disease.
	Tobacco smokings and/or coffee and tea drinking	Smoking may reduce the effectiveness considerably while drinking of tea or coffee may have same but smaller effects.
	Verapamil	Serious cardiodepression may occur by the concurrent use. Hence initial close supression and monitoring is recommended.
	X-ray contrast media	Hypotension is reported by concurrent use.

Calcium-channel blockers[1,2]

Drugs	Interaction with	Effects
Calcium-channel blockers	Aspirin	The antiplatelet effect of Ca-channel blockers may be increased by the concurrent use. Bruising is reported.
	Calcium salts	The effectiveness may be antagonized by the concurrent use.
	Cimetidine or ranitidine	Serum levels may be increased by cimetidine. Ranitidine interact minimally but famotidine appears to be reduce the heart activity.
	Dantrolene	Hyperkalaemia and cardiovascular collapse is reported.
	Food	Don't interact with clinical importance.
	Clonidine	Clonidine may provide additional effects.
	Local anaesthetics	Bradycardia and hypotension may occur by the concurrent use.
	Magnesium salts	Muscle weakness paralysis is reported by the concurrent use.
	Miscellaneous drugs	Concurrent use should be avoided to escape from the risk of the development of the torsodes depointes.
	Rifampicin	Serum levels may be reduced to that level making therapeutically ineffective if the dosage is not increased appropriately.
	Sulphinpyrazone	The clearance may be markedly increased.
	Vancomycin	The effectiveness may be increased by the concurrent use.
	X-ray contrast media	The hypotensive effects are increased by the presence of calcium-channel blockers. Ventricular tachycardia is reported by the concurrent use.

Oral Contraceptives and Related Sex Hormone Drugs[1,2]

Drugs	Interaction with	Effects
Oral contraceptives	Alcohol	Although blood alcohol remains unaltered, the detrimental effects may be reduced by the concurrent use.
	Antacids	A few evidence suggest the concurrent to be safe, but magnesium ticitrate may reduce the effects and reliability is also reported.
Oral contraceptives	Anti-asthmatic preparations	No recorded interaction is available. But asthmatic condition may be worsened and sometimes may be improved as well.
	Antibiotics and anti-infective agents	Concurrent use may lead to the failure of oral contraceptives to prevent pregnancy.
	Anticonvulsants	Concurrent use reports uncertainty towards action of oral contraceptives. Intermediate breakthrough bleeding, spotting and even pregnancies may occur. Sodium valproate does not interact.
	Antihypertensive agents	Anti-hypertensive agents appear resistant towards the hypertension caused by oral contraceptives.
	Cimetidine	Cimetidine may raise the serum oestradiol levels.
	Fluconazole	May reduce the effectiveness and even pregnancies may occur.
	Griseofulvin	Concurrent use may reduce the effects by the effects of oral contraceptives.

Contd...

Drugs	Interaction with	Effects
	Ketoconazole	May reduce the effectiveness of oral contraceptives by the concurrent use associated with intestinal bleeding.
	Penicillins	May cause the oral contraceptives to fail.
	Rifampicin	Concurrent use may cause the reliability of oral contraceptives uncertain.
	Tobacco smoking	May increase the rise of thromboembolic disease.
	Triacetyloleandomycin	Concurrent use may produce severe pruritis and jaundice.
	Vitamins	Oral contraceptives may rise the serum levels of vitamin A and lower levels of ascorbic acid, cyanocobalamin, folic acid and pyridoxin.
	Anti-inflammatory agents	Concurrent use may produce oceatin failure to prevent pregnancy.
	Aminoglutethimide	May reduce the serum levels markedly.
Intrauterine contraceptive diuretics (IUD's)	Aspirin, Codein, Paracetamol	Concurrent use may produce failure to prevent pregnancy.
	Mefenamic acid	Concurrent use may produce failure to prevent pregnancy.
Medroxyprogesterone	Aminoglutethimide	Aminoglutethimide markedly reduces the serum level of medroxyprogesterone.

Cytotoxic Drugs[1,2]

Drugs	Interaction with	Effects
Cytotoxic drugs	Aclarubicin	The effectiveness of aclarubicin can be increased.
Aminoglutethimide	Bendroflumethiazide	Prolong treatment with drug may cause serious loss of sodium.

Contd...

Drugs	Interaction with	Effects
Azathioprine/ Mereaptopurine	Allopurinol	Concurrent use may increase the effectiveness if cytotoxic agents is given orally. To avoid intoxication, dosage of cytotoxic drugs should be reduced to a third or a quarter. No interaction takes place on intravenous administration of cytotoxic drug.
	Cotrimoxazole or Trimethoprin	Concurrent use may increase the risk of life-threatening haematological toxicity.
	Doxorubicin (Adriamylin)	Concurrent use may increase the effectiveness.
Bleomycin	Cisplatin	Pulmonary toxicity of bleomycin is reported.
	Oxygen	Serious and fatal pulmonary toxcity can develop.
	Radiotherapy	Toxicity enhanced.
	Various cytotoxic regimens	The effectiveness, the bleomycin-induced pulmonary reactions in particular is increased by the concurrent use.
	Vincristin	Debilitation syndrome is produced.
Busulphan	Vaccination	Immunisation will live viruses can acuse life threatening infection.
	Thioguanine	Combination may results in nodular regenerative hyperplasia, portal hypertension, varices.
	Cyclophosphamide	Enhances haemopoietic therapeutic recovery.
Carmofur	Alcohol	A disulfiram-like reaction may occur.
Carmustine (BCNU)	Cimetidine	Concurrent use may increase the effectiveness but the fall in neutrophil and thrombocyte counts may become serious.

Contd...

Drugs	Interaction with	Effects
Chlorambucil	Myelosuppressive agents	Potentiation.
	Phenylbutazone and Warfarin	Effect of chlorambucil is potentiated.
Cisplatin	Aminoglycoside antibiotics	Potentiate neurotoxicity.
	Antihypertensive agents	Kidney failure by the concurrent use is reported.
Cisplatin	Ethacrynic acid	The effectiveness may be increased by the concurrent use.
	Ethacrynic acid	Fetal methotrexate toxicity may develop by the concurrent use.
	Probenecid	No report is available with certain support.
Cyclophosphamide	Allopurinol	Increased risk of bone-marrow toxicity.
	Benzodiazepines	Toxicity of cyclophosphamide may be increased by the concurrent use.
	Myelotoxic drug or radiotherapy	Serious toxicity is reported.
	Chloramphenicol	Increased risk of bone marrow toxicity.
	Corticosteroids	The effects may be reduced by the concurrent use.
	Dapsone	The effects may be reduced.
	Doxorubicin (Adriamycin)	Increased risk of cardiotoxicity.
	Morphine or Pethidine	The toxicity may be increased by the concurrent use.
	Phenobarbital	Metabolism & leukopenic activity increases.
Cyclophosphamide or Mustine	Sulphaphenazole	May increase or decrease the effects of cyclophosphamide.
Cyclophosphamide	Calcium channel blockers	The efficiency may be increased but reduction in absorption is reported.

Contd...

Drugs	Interaction with	Effects
Cytotoxic drugs	Food	Absorption may be reduced while other effects remain unaltered.
	Gentamycin	Hypomagnesaemia is reported by the concurrent use.
	Vaccines	The immune response of the body is suppressed by cytotoxic drugs. The effectiveness of vaccine may be poor.
Cytarabin	Radiotherapy & other myelotoxic Drugs	Bone marrow depression is potentiated.
Daunorubicin	Vaccination	Not recommended.
	Radiation	Enhanced radiation reaction.
	Heparin, Aluminum dexamethasone	Incompatable.
Doxorubicin (Adriamycin)	Actinomycin, Plicamycin, Methranycin	Concurrent use may cause fatal cardiomyopathy.
	Barbiturates	The current use may cause reduced effects.
	Mercaptopurine	Cholestasis induced by mercaptopurine may be potentiated by the drug.
	Beta-blockers	Cardiotoxicity is reported.
	Streptozotocin	Toxicity may be increased.
Etoposide	Cytotoxic Drugs	Synergism.
5-fluorouracil	Aminoglycosides	Gastrointestinal absorption may be delayed by the concurrent use.
	Cimetidine	Serum levels may be increased by 75%.
	Other bone marrow depressants and immuno-suppressive agents	Additive adverse effects.
	Vaccination	Simultaneous live viral vaccination may produce generalised and life threatening infection, killed virus vaccines are ineffective.

Contd...

Drugs	Interaction with	Effects
Hexamethylmelamine	Antidepressants	Severe orthoststic hypotension is reported.
Hydroxyurea	CNS depressants	Increased CNS depression is reported.
	Cytarabin	Risk of haematological toxicity increased.
I-fosfamide	Barbiturates	Encephalopathy is reported by the concurrent use.
	Cisplastin	Intoxication of ifosfamide may be increased.
	Warfarin	Effect of warfarin increased.
L-asparaginase	Methotrexate or cytarabin	Striking synergistic effect.
Leukovorin	Methotraxate	Reduces methotrexate activity.
	Fluorouracil	Enhance cytotoxic effect of fluorouracil.
Lomustine (CCNU)	Theophylline	Thrombocytopenia and bleeding is reported by concurrent use.
Melphalan	Cimetidine	Bioavailability of melphalan be reduced by the concurrent use.
Mercaptopurine	**Food**	The absorption is reduced and delayed by the concurrent use.
	Allopurinol	Effect drug enhanced by allopurinol.
	Hepatotoxic Drugs	Toxicity of mercaptopurine is potentiated.
	Myelosuppressive Drugs	Antineoplastic effect is potentiated.
	Warfarin	Anticoagulant effect of warfarin may be inhibited.
Methotrexate	Alcohol	Risk of hepatic cirrhosis and fibrosis may be increased.
	Amiodarone	Toxicity of methotrexate is reported by concurrent use.
	Aminoglycosides	Absorption may be reduced by the concurrent use of the paromomycin, neomycin and other oral aminoglycosides.

Contd...

Drugs	Interaction with	Effects
	Barbiturates	Alopecia caused by methotrexate may be increased by concurrent use.
	Chloramphenicol, PAS, Sodium Salicylate, Sulphomethoxy pyridazine, Tetracycline, Tolbutamide.	Intoxication may be enhanced by the concurrent use.
	Cholestyramine	The serum level can be markedly reduced by the concurrent use.
	Corticosteroids	The intoxication may be increased with the reduction of efficacy of methotrexate.
	Co-trimoxazole or Trimethoprine	Bone marrow depression and even fatal instances are reported.
	Diuretics	Concurrent use may reduce the bone-marrow supression.
	5-Flurouracil (5-FU)	The effectiveness may be reduced by the concurrent use.
	Nitrous oxide	Methotrexate induced stomatitis and other toxic effects may be enhanced by the concurrent use.
	Non-steroidal antiinflammatory drugs (NSAID's)	Concurrent use may cause rise in the serum levels and life threatening toxicity.
	Penicillins	The loss of methotrexate from the body may be reduced considerably by the concurrent use.
	Probenecids	Serum levels may be increased even by 3-4 folds by the concurrent use.
	Retinoids	Although concurrent use may be useful but toxic hepatitis is also reported.
	Teracyclins	Methotrexate intoxication may develop by the concurrent use.

Contd...

Drugs	Interaction with	Effects
	Urinary alkalinizers	May increase the solubility of methotrexate in urine but may increase its excretion.
	Salicylate, sulphonamides, phenytoin, phenylbutazone, tetracyclines, chloramphenicol, para-amino-benzoic acid	Toxicity of methotrexate increases.
Misonidazole	Cimetidine	Does not interact.
	Miscellaneous drugs	Clearance from the body may be increased by phenytoin, phenobarbitone, dexamethazone. Metoclpramide does not interact.
Mitomycin	Chlorozofocin	Pneumonitis by the concurrent use is reported.
	Adiramycin	Adiramycin induced cardiotoxicity is potentiated.
	Nitrosourea, Doxorubicine	Enhancement of pulmonary damage.
Mitozatrone	5-Flurouracil, Vincristin, Dacarbazine, Methotrexate	Synergistic affect.
Mustin HCI	Other mytotoxic and bone marrow suppressive drugs	Severe myelosuppression.
Procarbazine	CNS depressants or antihypertensives	The effectiveness may be increased by the concurrent use.
	Mustiline (Mechlorethamine, Nitrogen mustard)	Neurological toxicity may develop by the concurrent use.
	Tyramine-containing food and sympathomimetic amines	Itching skin reaction is reported by the concurrent use.
Streptozocin	Phenytoin	Concurrent use may reduce and even abolish the effectiveness.

Contd…

Drugs	Interaction with	Effects
Tamoxifen	Warfarin	Warfarin enhanced fatal results.
	Aminoglutethimide	Plasma Tamoxifen concentration reduced.
Vinblastin	Bleomycin, Cisplatin	Cardiovascular toxicity is reported.
Vinca alkaloids	Mitomycin	Pulmonary toxicity of mitomycin may be increased.
Vincristine	Colaspase, Isaoniazid and Pyridoxine	Concurrent use may increase the vincristine neurotoxicity.
	Mytomycin C	Acute bronchospasm.
	Other myelosuppressive Drugs	Potentiation.
	Digoxin	Serum digoxin level decreased.
	Methotrexate	Synergistic effect.

Digitalis Glycosides[1,2]

Drugs	Interaction with	Effects
Digitalis glycosides	ACE inhibitors	Serum levels may be raised up to 20-25% by the concurrent use. Enalapril, lisinopril and Ramipril appear not to interact.
	Amiloride	Amiloride may reduce the contractibility of heart by concurrent use.
	Aminoglutethimide	Concurrent use may increase the clearance of digitoxin.
	Aminosalicylic acid (PAS)	Concurrent use may reduce the blood levels of digitoxin.
	(Para)- Aminosalicylic acid (PAS)	No certain and important information is reported.
	Amiodarone	Concurrent use may make double the blood levels of digoxin. Dosage reduction is necessary to avoid digitalis intoxication.
	Amphotericin	Digitalis toxicity is reported.

Contd...

Drugs	Interaction with	Effects
	Antacids	Antacids may reduce the bioavailability of digoxin. A gap by 1-2 hr may be advised to avoid admixture in the gut.
	Azapropazone	Very occational small rise in blood level is reported.
	Barbiturates	Effectiveness is expected to be reduced by the concurrent use.
	Benzodiazepines	Digoxin intoxication and reduction in the urinary clearance is reported by the concurrent use.
	Beta-blockers	Concurrent use may cause bradycardia by the concurrent use.
	Clacium channel blockers	May rise the serum levels so dosage reduction is required.
	Calcium preparations	The concurrent use may enhance the effectiveness of digitalis and life threatening heart-arrhythmias may occur if intravenous calcium is administered.
	Carbamazepine	Bradycardia is reported by the concurrent use.
	Carbenoxolone	Carbenoxolone may raise blood pressure, disturb sodium-potassium level which may lead to congestive heart-failure.
	Cholestyramine	Reduction in serum levels for both are reported.
	Cimetidine	Rise or fall in serum levels are reported.
	Cisapride	May cause very small and clinically unimportant change in absorption.
	Colestipol	No interference in the absorption is reported.
	Cylosporin (e)	Kidney dysfunction and increased serum levels are reported by concurrent use.
	Cytotoxic (Antineoplastic) agents	Concurrent use may increase the absorption if digoxin is provided in fatal form.

Contd...

Drugs	Interaction with	Effects
	Dietary fibre (Bran) and laxatives	Dietary fibre in large amount and bulk-forming laxatives containing isphagula may have a significant effects on the absorption from the gut.
	Diltiazem	20-85% increase in the serum levels is reported by the concurrent use.
	Diuretics, potassium depleting agent	May cause increased digitalis toxicity.
	Edrophonium	Bradycardin and AV-block may occur by concurrent use.
	Enoximone	No change in serum level reported.
	Erythromycin, Tetracycline or other antibiotics	10% patients treated with erythromycin may show increment in serum level to double leading to digitalis intoxication.
	Enoldopam	Very small and unimportant change in serum levels is reported.
	Guanethidine and related drugs	No change in the effects is reported.
	Hydroxychloroquine and Chloroquine	70% increment in the serum levels is reported.
	Ibuprofen	Concurrent use may increase the serum levels by the concurrent use.
	Indomethacin	Serum levels may be increased up to 40% by the concurrent use. Dosage reduction is required to avoid intoxication.
	Kaolin-Pectin	Serum levels may be reduced. Taking dosage by 2 hr apart is advised to avoid interaction.
	Methyldopa	Bradycardia is reported by concurrent use.
	Metoclopramide	Metoclopramide interferes with absorption of solid dosage forms of digitalis glycosides.

Anti Hyperglycaemic Agents[1,2]

Drugs	Interaction with	Effects
Anti hyperglycaemic agents	ACE inhibitor	Concurrent use is reported to be uneventful.
	Alcohol	Delayed hypoglycaemia may occur if one drinks beyond moderation and accompanied by food.
	Allopurinol	Increment in the half life of chlorpropamide and decrease of tolbutamide is reported by the concurrent use.
	Amiloride	Hyperkalaemia may occur by the concurrent use.
	Anabolic steroids	The effects of the insulin may be reduced by the concurrent use.
	Anaesthetics	Extreme adverse effects is not reported. However for extensive surgical procedure, a change from oral antidiabetic treatment is advisable.
	Anticoagulants	Increased hypoglycaemia and anticoagulants effects is reported by the concurrent use of dicoumarol and tolbutamide.
	Azapropazone	Severe hypoglycaemia is reported by the concurrent use.
	Beta-blockers	Hypoglycaemia may occur and increased sweating is reported by the concurrent use.
	Calcium channel blockers	Calcium channel blockers are reported to have effects on insulin secretion and glucose regulation.
	Chloramphenicol	Concurrent use is reported to have increased hypoglycaemia.
	Chlorpromazine	Blood sugar may be increased by chlorpromazine and hence the dose of hypoglycaemic agent is required to be increased.

Contd...

Drugs	Interaction with	Effects
	Cimetidine or Ranitidine	Cimetidine or ranitidine may increase the effects of glipizile, gliclazide.
	Clofibrate	The effectiveness may be increased by clofibrate.
	Clonidine	May suppress the sign of hypoglycaemia in patients.
	Contraceptives (oral)	Oral contraceptives are reported to cause the dose of hypoglycaemic agents to be increased or decreased.
	Corticosteroids	The effects are opposed by corticosteroids.
	Cytotoxics	Control of diabetics may be severely disturbed by the concurrent use.
	Ethacrynic acid	May oppose the effects of hypoglycaemic action.
	Fenfluramine	May increase the effects.
	Frusemide	Increment in blood sugar.
	Guanethidine and related drugs	Increment in hypoglycaemic action is reported.
	Halofenate	May cause enhance blood sugar and lowering effects of chlorpropramide, tolbutamide tolazamide and phenformin.
	Heparin	Hypoglycaemia is reported by the concurrent use.
	Isoniazid	Raise of blood sugar by concurrent use.
	Lithium carbonate	May rise blood sugar by concurrent use.
	Methylsergide	The effectiveness of tolbutamide may be increased by the concurrent use.
	Miconazole	Hypoglycaemia is reported by the concurrent use.
	Monoamine oxidase inhibitors (MAOI)	Concurrent use may enhance the effectiveness.

Contd...

Drugs	Interaction with	Effects
	Non-steroidal antiinflammatory drugs (NSAID's)	Severe hypoglycaemia is reported when fenclofenac is given with chlorpropamide and metformin. Ibuprofen may increase the effects of glipizide.
	Phenylbutazone	Phenylbutazone may increase the effectiveness.
	Phenylephrine	Elevated blood pressure is reported by the concurrent use.
	Phenyramidol	The effects may be increased.
	Probenecid	Clearance from the body may be prolonged.
	Quinine or Quinidine	Severe hypoglycaemia is reported by the concurrent use.
	Rifampicin	Rifampicin may reduce the serum levels by concurrent use.
Hypoglycaemic agents	Salicylates	Aspirin and other salicylates may reduce the blood sugar.
	Sugar-containing pharmaceuticals	Liquid antibiotics, cough linctuses, bulk laxatives may cause additional diabetic problems.
	Sulphin pyrazone	Severe hypoglycaemia may occur by concurrent use.
	Sulphonamides	Effects may be increased.
	Tetracyclines	Oxytetracycline may enhance the effects which is also similar with doxycycline.
	Thiazides, chlorthalidone or related diuretics	May reduce the effects of hypoglycaemic agents and hyponatraemia is also reported.
	Tobacco smoking	Smokers requires more insulin.
	Tricyclic antidepressants	Hypoglycaemia is reported.
	Urinary alkalinizers and acidifiers	The effects of chlorpropamide is decreased if urine is made alkaline and increased if urine is acidified but no adverse interaction is reported.

Immunosupressant Agents[1,2]

Drugs	Interaction with	Effects
Corticosteroids	Aminoglutethimide	The effects of dexamethasone may be reduced and even abolished by the concurrent use.
	Antacids	The absorption may be reduced by large.
	Anti-infective agents	Corticosteroids generally suppress the normal potential of the body to attack by micro organism, it is required to make sure that anti-infective agent is capable to prevent the threat of potential infection.
	Barbiturates	Concurrent use may decrease the effects by concurrent use and hence corticosteroids dosage may require to be increased.
	Caffeine	Falsified information may be provided.
	Carbamazepine	The loss from the body may be increased by concurrent use.
	Carbimazole or Methimazole	The loss of prednisolone from the body may be increased. Hence its dosage is required to be increased.
	Cimetidine or Ranitidine	Cimetidine or Ranitidine appears not to interact.
	Contraceptives (Oral)	Oral contraceptives may increase the serum levels by concurrent use.
	Diuretics, Potassium losing	Concurrent use may cause excessive loss of potassium from the body which may lead to depletion. So, intake of potassium should be increased to balance the loss.

Contd...

Drugs	Interaction with	Effects
	Ephedrine	Dexamethasone loss from the body is enhanced by ephedrine while other does not interact.
	Ketoconazole	May reduce the absorption by concurrent use.
	Macrolide	May show higher toxic effects.
	Non-steroidal antiinflammatory drugs (NSAID's)	Gastrointestinal bleeding and ulceration may occur by concurrent use.
	Phenytoin	The effects may be reduced by concurrent use.
	Primidone	The effectiveness may be reduced by primidone by concurrent use.
	Rifampicin (Rifampin)	Rifampicin may reduce the effects by concurrent use.
	Live vaccines	Life threatening infections may occur by concurrent use.
Cyclosporins	Aminoglycosides antibiotics	Kidney toxicity may be enhanced by concurrent use.
	Amphotericine B	Kidney toxicity may be enhanced by concurrent use.
	Anticoagulants	May increase the need of higher dose of the both by concurrent use.
	Anticonvulsants	Serum levels may be reduced by concurrent use and 2-3 folds increase in the dosage may be needed.
	Calcium channel blockers	Cyclosporin serum levels may be enhanced.
Cyclosporin	Cholestyramin and food	Absorption may be affected by concurrent use.
	Corticosteroids	Convulsion is reported by the concurrent use.
	Diuretics	Concurrent use may cause nephrotoxicity.

Contd...

Drugs	Interaction with	Effects
	Etoposide	May be effective in the leukaemia treatment but severe side effect is reported.
	Fluconazole, Itraconazole, Ketoconazole	5-10 fold rise in serum level may occur if ketoconazole is used concurrently. A small rise is observed with the other two.
	Macrolide and related antibiotics	Marked rise in serum levels is reported by the concurrent use leading to cyclosporin toxicity. Dosage reduction is required.
	Metoclopramide	May increase the absorption increasing the serum levels.
	Non-steroidal antiinflammatory drugs (NSAID's)	Nephrotoxicity is reported by the concurrent use.
	Octreolide	Sharp fall in serum levels is reported.
	Probucol	Serum level reduction is reported.
Cyclosporine	Rifampicin	Sharp and marked fall in serum level is reported if dosage is increased by 2-3 folds.
	Sex hormones and related drugs	Hepatotoxicity is reported when used with oral contraceptives.
Cyclosporin	Sulphonamides, trimethoprin or Cotrimoxazole	Renal disfunction is reported by concurrent use. Drastic fall in serum level may on when both given intravenously.
	Vaccines	May cause immunity deficiency when given with influenza vaccine.

Lithium Drug Interaction[1,2]

Drugs	Interaction with	Effects
Lithium carbonate	ACE inhibitors	Lithium toxicity is reported by the concurrent use.
	Acetazolamide, Chlormerodrin, Spironolactone, Triamterene	Excretion of may be increased by triamterene and acetazolamide. Lithium intoxication is also reported.
	Baclofen	Huntington's chorea showed aggregation by the concurrent use.
	Calcium channel blockers	Increase in the effects, lithium intoxication and decrease in serum levels is reported. Bradycardia is also reported.
	Carbamazepine	Neurotoxicity is reported by the concurrent use.
	Cisplantin	Fall in serum levels with no clinical importance is reported.
	Co-trimoxazole	Lithium intoxication is reported by concurrent use.
	Diazepam	Hypothermis may develop by the concurrent use.
	Fluoxetine	Lithium toxicity is reported by concurrent use.
	Frusemide or Bumetamide	Although concurrent use is reported to be safe, but serious lithium intoxication is also reported.
	Haloperidol	Adverse reaction is reported by the concurrent use.
	Iodides	Additional hypothyroidic and goitrogenic effects are reported.
	Isphagula husk	Reduced serum level is reported by the concurrent use.
	Low sodium diet	Can increase tubular reabsorption of lithium and cause increased toxicity.
	Mazindol	Lithium intoxication is reported by the concurrent use.
	Methyldopa	Lithium intoxication is reported by the concurrent use.
	Metronidazole	Concurrent use reports rise in serum levels.

Contd...

Drugs	Interaction with	Effects
	Non-steroidal antiinflammatory drugs (NSAID's)	60% rise in serum levels is reported with clometacin and Indomethacin whereas around 15-34% rise with diclofenac and ibuprofen is reported.
	Phenytoin	Concurrent use may cause lithium intoxication.
	Sodium chloride or bicarbonate	May rise the serum levels and ingesion of sodium may prevent the maintenance of lithium serum levels.
	Spectinomycin	Concurrent use may cause intoxication.
	Tetracycline	Lithium intoxication is reported by concurrent use.
	Theophylline	Reduced serum level by 20-30% is reported by the concurrent use.
	Thiazides or related diuretics	Serum levels may be increased leading to lithium intoxication.

Monoamine Oxidase Inhibitors[1,2]

Drugs	Interaction with	Effects
Monoamine oxidase inhibitor	Amantadine	An isolated report describes a rise in blood pressure in a patient on amantadine when given phenelzine.
	Barbiturates	Generally MAOI can enhance and prolong the activity of the barbiturates but a few isolated report describes an interaction in man.
	Benzodiazepines	Concurrent use may cause adverse effects like oedema, chorea.
	Chloral hydrate	Fatal hyper-pyrexia is reported by the concurrent use.
	Cyproheptadine	Hallucination is reported by the concurrent use.
	Dextropmethorphan	Hyperpyrexia may be occurred by the concurrent use.

Contd...

Drugs	Interaction with	Effects
	Dextropropoxyphene	Increament in the sedative effect is reported by the concurrent use.
	Fenfluramine	Concurrent use is effective.
	Ginseng	Adverse effects are reported by the concurrent use.
	Mazindol	Increase in the blood level is reported by the concurrent use.
	Methyldopa	Delayed development of hallucinosis is reported. The order of administration is reported to be important.
	Monoamine oxidase inhibitor	Stroke and hypertensive reaction is reported by the concurrent use.
	Morphine or Methadone	Hypotension is reported although very rare.
	Oxtriphylline	Tachycardia and apprehension may be occurred by concurrent administration.
	Phenothiazine	Fatal reaction with methotrimeprazine is reported.
	Rauwolfia alkaloids or tetrabenazine	Central association with hypertension may occur if MAOI is administered first.
	Sulphonamides	Weakness, ataxia and other adverse effects may occur by concurrent use.
	Tricyclic antidepressants	Concurrent use is contraindicacious. However extreme careful monitoring may bring advantageous result.
	L – tryptophan	Neurological sign of toxicity is reported by concurrent use.

Neuroleptic, Anxiolytic and Tranquilizing Drugs[1,2]

Drugs	Interaction with	Effects
Benzodiazepines	Antacids	The absorption may be delayed by concurrent use with antacids.
	Beta-blockers	Patients on diazepam may be more accident prone while taking beta-blockers.
	Cimetidine, Ranitidine, Famotidine, Nizatidine	Except cimetidine, no interaction is reported with others. Serum levels may be raised by cimetidine. Dose of alprazolam should be reduced to 1/3 rd when administered concurrently with cimetidine.
	Contraceptives, Oral	Oral contraceptives may raise the effectiveness of alprazolam, chlordiazepoxide diazepam, nitrazepam & triazolam but reduction in effects of oxazepam, lorazepam and temazepam are reported.
Benzodiazepines	Desipramide	Alprazolam enhances the activity of desipramide.
	Dextropropoxyphene	Serum levels may be raised by concurrent use.
	Disulfiram	Serum levels may be increased leading to drowsiness is reported.
	Ethambutol	No interaction is reported by the concurrent use.
	Imipramine	Alprazolam enhances the activity of imipramine.
	Indomethacin	No adverse effects is reported except increament in the filling of dizziness.
	Isoniazid	Reduces the loss from the body. Increase in the effect of diazepam & triazolam is expected. No interaction is reported with oxazepam or clotiazepam.

Contd...

Drugs	Interaction with	Effects
	Lithium	May produce hypothermia in case of diazepam.
	Macrolide antibiotics	Erythromycin, triacetyloleandomycin and Josamycin may alter the serum level to higher side. Hence dosage reduction may be necessary.
	MAOls	Potentiate action of diazepam and lorazepam.
	Omeprazole	Clearance from the body may be delayed. Prolongation of clobazam action is reported.
	Probenecids	May reduce the loss from the body thus higher sedative effects may be expected.
	Rifampicin (Rifampin)	May cause marked increase in the loss from the body.
	Theophylline and caffeine	Caffeine may reduce the sedative effects.
	Tobacco smoking	Smokers may require larger doses than the non-smokers.
	Valproate	May increase plasma clobazam concentration.
Buspirone	Fluoxetine	Concurrent use may reduce the effects of buspirone.
Droperidol/Hyoscine	Monoamine oxidase inhibitors (MAOI)	Hypotension is reported by concurrent use.
Haloperidol	Alcohol	CNS depressant effects enhanced.
	Antituberculars	The serum levels of haloperidol may be reduced by concurrent use.
Haloperidol	Carbamazepine	Neurotoxicity is reported during concurrent use. Reduce plasma concentration.
	Fluoxetine	Development of extrapyramidol symptoms is reported by concurrent use.
	Guanrthidine	Guanethidine effect may be decreased.

Contd...

Drugs	Interaction with	Effects
	Lithium	Increases lithium blood levels and may predispose to neuroleptic malignant syndrome.
	Metoclopramide	Adverse effect may be increased.
	Indomethacin	Confusion and drowsiness is reported by concurrent use.
	Rifampicin	Plasma concentration may be reduced by concurrent administration.
	Tobacco smoking	Smokers require more doses than nonsmokers.
	Tricyclic antidepressants	Increases adverse effects of tricyclic antidepressants.
Hydroxyzine	Alcohol	Potentiates CNS depression.
	Barbiturates	Potentiates CNS depression.
	Opoid analgesic	Potentiates CNS depression.
	Monoamine oxidase	Potentiates antimuscarinic effects.
	Atropine	Potentiates antimuscarinic effects.
	Tricyclic antidepressants	Potentiates antimuscarinic effects.
	Aminophylline	Incompatibility with hydroxyzine.
	Chloramphenicol	Incompatibility with hydroxyzine.
	Benzylpenicillin	Incompatibility with hydroxyzine.
	Miscellaneous drugs	High dose of hydroxyzine may cause ECG abnormalities.
Neuroleptics (Butyrophenones, Phenothiazines, Thioxazthenes)	Anticholinergics	Mainly uneventful but occasional life-threatening reaction may occur.
	Bromocriptine	Concurrent use though mainly successful but re-emergence of schizophrenic symptoms is also reported.

Contd...

Drugs	Interaction with	Effects
Phenothiazines	Antacids	Antacids may reduce the serum levels.
	Antimalarials	Serum levels of phenothiazines may be enhanced.
	Ascorbic acid	Serum levels may be reduced is reported by concurrent use.
	Attapulgib	Fall in absorption is reported.
	Barbiturates	Presence of one reduces the other in serum levels.
	Cimetidine	Serum levels may be reduced by a third by concurrent use.
	Disulfiram	Re-emergence of psychotic symptoms is reported by concurrent use.
	Lithium carbonate	Extra-pyramidal side effects or neurotoxicity has been reported by the concurrent use.
	Naltrexone	Lethargy occurrence is reported by the concurrent use.
	Phebnylpropanolamine	Concurrent use may cause ventricular fibrillation.
	Tricyclic antidepressants	Mutual interaction is reported which causes rise in the serum levels of both drugs.
Sulpiride	Antacids or sucralfate	The absorption of sulpiride may be reduced by concurrent use.
Tetrabenazine	Chlorpromazine	Parkinson – like symptoms are reported by concurrent use.
	Haloperide	Can cause severe dopamine deficiency.
	Metoclopramide	Can cause severe dopamine deficiency.
Zolpidem	Alcohol	Enhances sedative action.
	Refampicin	Significantly reduces the plasma concentration and effect of zolpidem.
	Haloperidol	The effectiveness of haloperidol may be increased.
	Smoking	Heavy smoking may also reduces the effects.

Neuromuscular Blocker & Anaesthetic Drugs[1,2]

Drugs	Interaction with	Effects
Anaesthetics	Adrenaline, Noradrenaline and Terbutaline	Heart arrhythmias may develop by concurrent use unless control of dosage is not monitored.
	Alcohol	Who regularly drinks require higher dosage than those who donot drink.
	Anaesthetics	Myoclonic Seizures is reported by concurrent use.
	Antibiotics	The effectiveness may be increased by the concurrent use with aminoglycoside antibiotics.
	Antihypertensives	The normal homeostatic response of the cardiovascular system may be impaired.
	Beta – blockers	Concurrent use appears to be safe excepting methoxyflurane, cyclopropane, diethyl-ether, trichloroehylene.
	Calcium channel blockers	Impaired myocardial conduction is reported by concurrent use.
Anaesthetics	Fenfluramine	Cardiac arrest of fatal nature is attributed by concurrent use.
	Monoamine oxidase inhibitors	MAOI should be withdrawn well before anaesthesia is generally advised. In most cases it seems unnecessary. Though hypo and hypertension is reported by the concurrent use.
	Neuromuscular blockers	Nitrous oxide is reported to be noninteractive. Others inhalation anaesthetics may increase neuromuscular blockers.
	Phyrnylephrine	Phenylephrine eye drops may cause cyanosis and bradycardia.
Anaethetics (Metroxyflurane)	Phenytoin or Phenobarbitone	Phenytoin intoxication, hepatic necrosis are reported by concurrent use.

Contd...

Drugs	Interaction with	Effects
Anaesthetics and/or Neuromuscular blockers	Theophylline	Cardiac arrhythmias are reported by concurrent use.
	Tricyclic antidepressants	Tachyarrhythmias have been reported by concurrent use.
Anaesthetics (Local)	Alcohol and antirheumatics	Person who receives anti-rheumatic drugs and drinks may practice increased chances of failure rate of spinal anaesthesia.
	Anaesthetics (local)	Normally combined use is safe. However increased toxicity is supposed to be occured.
	Benzodiazepines	Conflicting evidence is reported about wheather diazepam can increase or decrease the concentration in the serum levels.
	Beta-blockers	Propanolol reduced the clearance of bupivacaine.
Neuromuscular blockers and/or Anaesthetic	Cimetidine or Ranitidine	Both cimetidine and ranitidine are reported to raise bupivacaine levels.
Neuromuscular blockers	Aminoglycoside antibiotics	Having neuromuscular blocking activity, aminoglycoside antibiotics should be appropriately measured to accommodate the increased neuromuscular blockade and prolonged fatal respiratory depression.
	Aprotinin	Apnoea is reported by concurrent use.
	Benzodiazepines	The effectiveness of neuromuscular blockers may be enhanced.
	Beta-blockers	Bradycardia and hypotension is reported. May increase or decrease in the extent of neurovascular blockade.
	Calcium channel blocker	Increased and prolonged neurovascular blockade is reported by the concurrent use.
	Carbamazepine	Carbamazepine reduces the time of recovery from neurovascular blockade.

Contd...

Drugs	Interaction with	Effects
	Cimetidine or Ranitidine	Ranitidine appears not to interact. Cimetidine however enhance the recovery time from neurovascular blockade.
	Cyclophosphamide	The effects may be enhanced and prolonged by concurrent use with cyclophosphamide.
	Cyclosporine	The effectiveness may be increased by concurrent use.
	Dantrolene	The muscle relaxant effects of dantrolene can be additive.
	Dexpanthenol	The effects may be increased by concurrent use.
	Ecothiopate iodide	The effects may be increased and prolonged.
	Fentanyl citrate-droperidol (innovar)	The effects may be prolonged by concurrent use.
	Frusemide	Lower doses of frusemide increases the effects, higher doses oppose the effectiveness.
	Immunosupresants	The effects may be reduced even by 2 to 4 folds by concurrent use.
	Insecticides	The neuromuscular blocking effects may be enhanced.
	Lignocaine, procaine or Procainamide	The effectiveness may be enhanced and prolonged by concurrent use.
	Lithium carbonate	Normally safe. However prolonged blockade and respiratory difficulties are also reported.
	Magnesium salts	The effects may be increased and prolonged by concurrent use.
	Metoclopramide	Increament and prolongation in the effects is reported by concurrent use.
	Miscellaneous antibiotics	Antibiotics having neuromuscular blocking activity should be appropriately measured to accommodate increased blockade. Metronidazole, Chloramphenicol, Penicillin is reported not to interact.
	Monoamine oxidase inhibitor	Concurrent use may enhance the effectiveness.

Contd...

Drugs	Interaction with	Effects
Neuromuscular blockers & anaesthetics	Morphine	Hypertension and tachycardia are reported by concurrent use.
Neuromuscular blockers	Phenytoin	Phenytoin may reduce the effects of most drugs except tubocurarine where the effect is minimum and atracurium with no interaction.
	Promazine	Apnoea is reported by concurrent use.
	Quinidine	Quinidine may enhance the effects of both depolarizing and nondepolarizing type. Recurarization and apnoea are reported.
	Quinine	Recurarization and apnoea are reported by concurrent use.
	Testosteron	Interference to the effects is reported.
	Thiotepa	Increament of effects are expected.
	Trimetaphan	The effects may be enhanced to prolonged apnoea.

Sympathomimetic Drugs[1,2]

Drugs	Interaction with	Effects
Amphetamines and related drugs	Chlorpromazine	The effects of both are opposed by one another.
Amphetamines	Lithium Carbonate	The effects are likely to be opposed by lithium carbonate.
	Nasal decongestants	Antagonism of I-amphetamine is reported.
	Urinary acidifiers or alkalinizers	Acidifiers increases the loss in the urine while it is reported being reduced by alkalinizers.
Directly acting sympathomimetics	Beta-blockers	Life-threatening hypertensive reaction resulting due to increament in the pressure effects of adrenalin may lead to bradycardia. Anaphylaxis is reported to be enhanced by concurrent use.

Contd...

Drugs	Interaction with	Effects
Directly or indirectly acting sympathomimetic amines	Furazolidone	Concurrent use may raise the blood pressure seriously.
Directly acting sympathomimetics	Guanethidine and related drugs	The pressure effects may be increased even by 2-4 folds by concurrent use.
	Mianserin or Trazodone	Generally no adverse effect is found. However toxicity on trazodone by pseudoephedrine is reported.
	Monoamine oxidase inhibitor (MAOI)	Moderate increment in the effects is reported.
Directly and indirectly acting sympathomimetics	Rauwolfia alkaloids	Slight increment in the effects is reported by rauwolfia alkaloids. The effects of indirectly acting or mixed activity may be even abolished.
Directly acting sympathomimetic amines	Tricyclic antidepressants	Hypertension, cardiac arrhythmias are reported to injection of noradrenalin and to a lesser extent to phenylephrine.
Dopamine	Ergometrine	Development of gangrene is reported by concurrent use.
	Phenytoin	Serious hypotension is reported by concurrent use.
Indirectly acting sympathomimetic amines	Methyldopa	No serious interaction is reported. Methyldopa however may depress the effects.
	Monoamine oxidase inhibitor (MAOI)	Hypertensive abnormalities and cricis are reported by concurrent use.
3, 4, – methylene-dioxymethamphetamine (MDMA)	Monoamine oxidase inhibitor (MAOI)	Hypertoxicity, altered mental status are reported by concurrent use.
Phenylpropanolamine	Indomethacin	Concurrent use of a single dose of indomethacin reported to develop serious hypertension.
Phenylephrine	Monoamine oxidase inhibitor (MAOI)	Concurrent use may lead to even life-threatening crisis.

Theophylline and Related Xanthine Drug Interactions [1,2]

Drugs	Interaction with	Effects
Theophylline	Allopurinol	Concurrent use may enhance the effects of theophylline.
	Aminoglutethimide	Theophylline loss from the body may be increased.
	Barbiturates	Theophylline serum level can be reduced.
	BCG vaccine	The theophylline serum levels may be increased by small extent.
	Beta-antagonist bronchodilators	No adverse interaction is reported. Due to side effect, hypokalaemia may occur.
	Beta-blockers	Bronchospasm may occur by concurrent use.
	Ephedrine	Chronic concurrent treatment increases adverse effects.
	Sympathomimetics	Cardiac arrhythmias (especially with preexsisting cardiac disease) may develop with concurrent use.
	Pancuronium	Tachycardia may develop with concurrent use.
	Cimetidine	Inhibition of metabolism is found with concurrent use.
	Propanolol	Inhibition of metabolism is found with concurrent use.
	Halothan	Potentiate cardiac arrythmias.
	Erythromycin	Reduce clearance.
	Phenobarbitone	Induces metabolism & clearance.
	Phenytoin	Induces metabolism & clearance.
	Rifampicin	Induces metabolism & clearance.
	Sulphinpyrazone	Enhances clearance.
Caffeine	Cimetidine	The stimulant effects of caffeine are increased by concurrent use.
	Oral contraceptives	The effects of caffeine may be enhanced by concurrent use.
	Disulfirum	The caffeine loss from the body may be reduced complicating the withdrawal from alcohol is reported.

Contd...

Drugs	Interaction with	Effects
	Idrocilamide	Retention time of caffeine in the body may be increased, resulting intoxication which may lead to insomnia, nervousness, anxious agitation.
	Methoxsalen	Loss of caffeine from the body may be reduced thus increases the possibility of caffeine intoxication.
	Mexiletine	30-60% reduction in caffeine clearence from the body is reported by concurrent use.
	Quinolone antibiotics	Enoxacin and pipemidic acid may increase the blood levels.
Theophylline	Erythromycin	Reduces clearance.
	Food	The bioavailability of theophylline from many preparation may be increased or decreased.
	Frusemide	Potentiate cardiac arrythmias.
	Halothane	Frusemide may increase, decrease or may be noninteractive.
	Idrocalamide	Theophylline levels may be increased.
	Influenza vaccine	Toxicity is reported in few patients by concurrent use.
	Interferon	Interferon reduces the clearance of theophylline from the body.
	Isoniazid	Concurrent use may increase the theophylline serum levels.
	Ketoconazole	May reduce theophylline levels in asthmatics.
	Macrolide antibiotics	Triacetylolcandomycin may raise theophylline serum levels.
	Mexilatine	Increased theophylline level and intoxication is reported.
Theophylline & related drugs	Probenecid	Serum theophylline level remain unaltered but diprophylline and enprofylline levels can be raised.
	Pyrantel	Increased serum theophylline level is reported.

Contd...

Drugs	Interaction with	Effects
	Quinolone antibiotics	Enoxacin or ciprofloxacin may raise serum theophylline level markedly. Nonfloxacin, lomefloxacin.
	Quinolone antibiotics	Ofloxacin and pefloxacin may cause to less extent.
	Rifampicin	Serum theophylline levels may be reduced.
	Sucralfate	Absorption of sustained release theophylline is reduced by sucralfate.
	Sulphinpyrazone	Serum theophylline levels may be reduced to small extent.
	Tetracycline or Cephalosporine	No adverse interaction of clinical importance is reported.
Theophylline	Thiabendazole	Serum theophylline levels may be significantly increased by concurrent use leading to theophylline intoxication.
	Thyroid & antithyroid compounds	Serum theophylline levels may be increased leading to intoxication.
	Ticlopidine	Clearance of theophylline from the body may be reduced.
	Tobacco smoking	Smokers may require more theophylline dose to obtain the desired effects.
	Vidarabine	Concurrent use may cause increase in the serum theophylline levels.
	Viloxazine	The serum theophylline levels may be increased by concurrent use leading to theophylline intoxication.

Tricyclic Antidepressants & Related Drug Interactions[1,2]

Drugs	Interaction with	Effects
	Cimetidine	Concurrent use may raise the femoxetine serum levels by 140%.
Femoxetine	Miscellaneous drugs	No adverse reaction is reported by concurrent use.
	Monoamine oxidase inhibitors (MAOI)	Serious reaction occur with concurrent use.

Contd...

Drugs	Interaction with	Effects
	Antidepressants	Two-fold increase in plasma levels of other antidepressants when concurrently use with fluoxetine.
	Diazepam	Half life of diazepam is prolonged.
	Warfarin	May cause transient shift in plasma concentration of warfarin resulting in adverse effects.
	Digoxin	May cause transient shift in plasma concentration of digoxin resulting in adverse effects.
Fluoxetine	L – Tryptophan	Concurrent use may cause central & peripheral toxicity.
Mianserin or Nomifensine	Anticonvulsants	Serum levels of both may be reduced by concurrent use.
Tetracyclic antidepressants	Beta-blockers	Maprotiline toxicity is reported by concurrent use.
Trazodone	Phenothiazine	Hypotension is reported by concurrent use.
Tricyclic antidepressants	MAOls	Dangerous combination. Trazodone should not be given within 2 weeks of discontinuing drug 76 Multiple sclerosis is reported.
	Baclofen	
	Barbiturates	
	Benzodiazepines	The serum levels may be reduced by the concurrent use of barbiturates.
	Cannabis	Drowsiness, forgetfulness are reported by concurrent use.
	Carbamazepine	Tachycardia is reported on smoking cannabis.
		Carbamazepine intoxication is reported by concurrent use.
Tricyclic antidepressants	Cholestyramine	Marked reduction in serum doxepine level is reported.
	Cimetidine or Ranitidine	Serum amitriptyline, desipramine, dexepin, imipramine, nortriptyline levels can be raised by concurrent use.

Contd...

Drugs	Interaction with	Effects
Tricyclic and related antidepressants	Co-trimoxazole	The symptoms may be relapsed by concurrent use.
Tricyclic antidepressants	Dextropropoxyphene	Increased lethargy and day time sedation is reported.
	Disulfirum	Disulfirum reduces the clearance from the body. The increament in the effects is reported.
	Ethchlorvynol	Concurrent use may cause transient delerium.
	Fenfluramine	A confusing situation is reported.
Tricyclic and related antidepressants	Fluoxetine	Serum desipramine, imipramine, nortriptyline and trazodone is increased by concurrent use.
Tricyclic antidepressants	**Food**	No effect in the absorption is reported.
	Furazolidone	Development of toxic psychosis, hyperactivity, sweating is reported by concurrent use.
	Haloperidol	Serum level of tricyclic antidepressants may be increased by concurrent use.
	Methadone	Serum levels may be doubled by methadone.
	Methylphenidate	Clinical improvement may be caused by concurrent use.
Tricyclic antidepressants	Oestrogens (estrogens)/oral contraceptives	The effects of imipramine may be reduced by oestrogens.
	Quinidine	Quinidine may reduce the losses of nortriptyline.
	Sucralfate	Absorption of amitriptyline is reduced by concurrent use.
	Thyroid preparations	Peroxysomal atrial tachycardia, thyrotoxicosis are reported by concurrent use.

Contd...

Drugs	Interaction with	Effects
	Tobacco smoking	Serum amitriptyline, clomipramine, desipramine, imipramine and nortriptyline levels may be reduced. However, free and unbound antidepressants may offset the effects of interaction.

Miscellaneous Drug Interactions[1]

Drugs	Interaction with	Effects
Acipimox	Cholestyramine	No significant interaction is reported.
Allopurinol	Antacids	Aluminum hydroxide antacid may reduce the effects.
	Iron	No adverse reaction is reported.
	Probenecid	No adverse interaction is reported.
	Tamoxifen	Concurrent use may cause marked enhancement in the effects of allopurinol.
	Thiazides	Renal failure and allergic reactions are attributed by concurrent use.
Anistreptase (APSAC)	Streptokinase	The effects of streptokinase may be reduced or even abolished.
Anticholinesterases	Miscellaneous drugs	Acetazolamide may oppose the actions. Dipuridamole, procainamide and quinidines also appear to oppose the action of drug used for myasthenia.
Antihistamines	Contraceptives, (oral)	No adverse reaction is reported.
Baclofen	Ibuprofen	Baclofen intoxication is reported by concurrent use.
Benzbromarone	Miscellaneous drugs	No confirmed interaction is reported.
Bismuth sublitrate	Miscellaneous drugs	Large amount of milk, antacids and food may reduce the effects.
Calcium &Vitamin D	Diuretics	Excessive serum calcium and Vitamin D levels may develop & urinary excretion of calcium can be reduced.

Contd...

Drugs	Interaction with	Effects
Cannabis	Disulfirum	Hypomanic-like reaction is reported by concurrent use.
Carbenoxolone	Antacids	The effectiveness may be reduced by antacids.
	Antihypertensives and diuretics	Carbenoxolone may cause flide retension and BP may be raised. Hypokalaemia is reported by the concurrent use of thiazide and carbenoxolone.
	Chlorpromide, Tolbutamide, Phenytoin, Warfarin.	Only chlorpromide is reported to cause a small reduction in serum carbenoxolone levels.
Charcoal	Other drugs	Charcoal may absorbs drugs into its surface and thus reduce the availability of drugs for absorption by gut.
Chlormethiazole (clomethiazole)	Cimetidine or Ranitidine	Ranitidine appears not to interact while cimetidine is reported to cause increament of the effectiveness.
Cholestyramine	Spironolactone	Concurrent use may cause hyperchloraimic metabolic acidosis.
Cisapride	Miscellaneous drugs	Cisapride may increase the rate of absorption of diazepam and alcohol.
Clofibrate	Cholestyramine	No sigificant interaction is reported.
	Contraceptives, oral	Oral contraceptives may raise the serum cholesterol and triglyceride.
	Probenecids	Probenecids may increase the serum clofibrate levels to double.
CNS depressants	CNS depressants	Life threatening consequences may occur by concurrent use.
Colestipol	Clofibrate or Fenofibrate	No adverse interaction is reported.
	Miscellaneous drugs	No interaction with aspirin or methyldopa. Interaction is reported in insulin-treated diabetics but is inert to those treated with phenformine and sulphonylurea.

Contd...

Drugs	Interaction with	Effects
Dimethicone	Cimetidine or doxycyclin	The bioavailability remains unaffected by dimethicone.
Dinoprostone (Prostaglandin E2)	Oxytocin	Uterine hypertonus is reported by concurrent use.
Enteral tube feeding	Antacids	Obstruction plug is reported with aluminium containing antacids.
Ergot	Glyceryl trinitrate (GTN)	Ergot is reported to oppose the effects of glyceryl trinitrate.
	Macrolide antibiotics	Ergot toxicity is reported by concurrent use with erythromycin or triacetyloleandomycin. No interaction occurs with midecanycin or spiramycin.
	Tetracyclins	Ergotism is reported by concurrent use.
Ethylenedibromide	Disulfirum	Concurrent use may cause malignant tumours in man so it is advised to avoid such use.
Famotidine, Nizatidine, Roxatidine	Other drugs	No adverse effect of clinical importance is reported.
Fenfluramine	Mazindol	Cardiomyopathy is reported by concurrent use.
Folic acid	Sulphasalazine	Absorption of folic acid may be reduced by concurrent use.
Gemfibrosil	Colestipol	Gemfibrozil absorption may be reduced.
	Ispaghula (Psyllium)	No important interaction is reported.
	Rifampicin	No interaction is reported.
Glucagon	Beta-blocker	The effects of glucagon may be reduced.
Glyceryl trinitrate (GTN)	Anticholinergics	Patients having such drugs reported to have dry mouth.
Glyceryl trinitrate (GTN)	Aspirin	GTN serum levels may be enhanced resulting side-effects like hypotension and headaches.

Contd...

Drugs	Interaction with	Effects
H$_2$ Blockers	Antacids	The absorption of cimetidine, ranitidine and famotidine may be reduced by antacids.
	Sucralfate	The healing rate may be increased by concurrent use.
	Tobacco smoking	Healing rate is less in smokers.
Iron preparations	Antacids	The absorption of iron may be reduced by concurrent use.
Iron or Vitamin B$_{12}$	Chloramphenicol	Fatal bone marrow depression, reversible depression are reported.
Iron preparation	Cholestyramine	Absorption may be reduced.
	Tea	No alteration in the absorption is reported.
Liquorice	Other drugs	Pseudoaldosteronism is reported by concurrent use.
Loperamide	Cholestyramine	The effectiveness of loperanide may be reduced.
Methoxalen	Phenytoin	Phenytoin may reduce the serum methoxsalen levels.
Metyrapone	Phenytoin	The effects of metyrapone may be reduced.
Oxygen (Hyperberic)	Acetazolamide, Barbiturates, Narcotics	Oxygen-induced convulsions are reported.
Paraldehyde	Disulfiram	To get rid of toxicity, concurrent use should be avoided.
Piperine	Miscellaneous drugs	Bioavailability of phenytoin and other drugs are increased.
Pirenzepine	Cimetidine	Pirenzepine increases the cimetidine-induced reduction in gastric acid secretion.
Pravestatin	Miscellaneous drugs	Bioavailability of pravestatin is reduced. No interaction with warfarin.
Retinoids	Tetracyclins, Vitamin A	Pseudotumour cerebri is reported to develop.
Roxatidine	Antacids and food	No interaction is reported.
Simvastatin	Miscellaneous drugs	No interaction is reported with beta-blockers, calcium antagonists, diuretics or NSAID's.

Contd…

Drugs	Interaction with	Effects
Sodium polystyrene sulphonate	Antacids	Metabolic alkalosis is reported.
	Sorbitol	Colonic necrosis may occur.
Somatropin (human growth hormone)	Miscellaneous hormones	Somatropin may reduce the effects of insulin and thyroid function.
Sulphinpyrazone	Flufenamic, Meclofenamic or Mefenamic acid	No adverse interaction is reported.
	Probenecid	Probenecid may reduce the loss in the urine.
Thyroid hormones	Anticonvulsants	Reduction in the effect of thyroxin is reported.
	Barbiturates	Reduction in the effect of thyroxin is reported.
	Cholestyramine	Concurrent use may reduce the absorption of thyroid extract, levothyroxin & triiodothyroxin.
Thyroid hormone	Levastatin	Rise in serum thyroid hormone levels is reported.
	Rifampicin (Rifampin)	The effects of thyroid hormone may be reduced.
Total parenteral nutrition	Potassium sparing diuretics	Metabolic acidosis is reported.
Trimoprostil	Antacids	No adverse interaction is reported.
Vitamin A	Aminoglycoside antibiotics	Absorption of vitamin A is reduced by meomycin.
Vitamin C (ascorbic acid)	Aspirin	The absorption of ascorbic acid is reduced by a third by concurrent use.
Vitamin D	Phenytoin	Osteomalacia is reported.
Vitamin K	Gentamycin and Clindamycin	Hypothrombinaemia is reported by concurrent use.
X-ray contrast media	Calcium channel blocker	The effects may be increased by calcium channel blockers. Tachycardia is reported.
	Cholestyramine	Poor radiographic visualization is reported.
	Phenothiazine	Epileptiform reaction is reported by concurrent use.

PART - B

HERB DRUG INTERACTION

Herbs are plant derived materials which are used for medicinal purpose. Herb-drug interactions are interactions that occur between herbal medicines and conventional drugs. These types of interactions may be more common than drug-drug interactions because herbal medicines often contain multiple pharmacologically active ingredients, while conventional drugs typically contain only one. Some such interactions are clinically significant, although most herbal remedies are not associated with drug interactions causing serious consequences. Most herb-drug interactions are moderate in severity. The most commonly implicated conventional drugs in herb-drug interactions are warfarin, insulin, aspirin, digoxin, and ticlopidine, due to their narrow therapeutic indices. The most commonly implicated herbs involved in such interactions are those containing St. John's Wort, magnesium, calcium, iron, or ginkgo. The possibility of drug interactions, direct toxicities, and contamination with active pharmaceutical agents are among the safety concerns about dietary and herbal supplements. Although there is a widespread public perception that herbs and botanical products in dietary supplements are safe, research has demonstrated that these products carry the same dangers as other pharmacologically active compounds. Interactions may occur between prescription drugs, over-the-counter drugs, dietary supplements, and even small molecules in food—making it a daunting challenge to identify all interactions that are of clinical concern.

Concerns about herb-drug interactions are often not based on rigorous research. Most herb-drug interactions identified in current sources are hypothetical, inferred from animal studies, cellular assays, or based on other indirect means; however, attention to this issue is needed for drugs with a narrow therapeutic index, such as cancer chemotherapeutic agents, warfarin, and digoxin.

To date, well-designed clinical studies evaluating herbal supplement-drug interactions are limited and sometimes inconclusive. This issue of the Digest provides information about several herbs and their potential interactions with other agents.

The mechanisms underlying most herb-drug interactions are not fully understood. Interactions between herbal medicines and anticancer drugs typically involve enzymes that metabolize cytochrome P450. For example, St. John's Wort has been shown to induce CYP3A4 and P-glycoprotein *in vitro* and *in vivo*.

TABLE 1

Herb-drug Interactions

Herbs	Drugs	Interaction
Scutellaria baicalensis	Losartan	May increase drug levels
	Rosuvastatin	May decrease drug levels
Berberis vulgaris	Drugs that displace the protein binding of bilirubin, e.g. phenylbutazone	May potentiate effect drug on displacing bilirubin
Vaccinlum myrtillus	Warfarin	Potentiation of bleeding
Cimicifuga racemosa	Statin drugs e.g.atorvastatin	May potentiate increase in liver enzymes, specifically ALT.
Fucus vesiculosus	Hyperthyroid medication, e.g. carbimazole	May decrease effectiveness of drug due to natural Iodine content
	Thyroid replacement therapies, e.g. thyroxine	May add to effect of drug.
Lycopusvirginicus, Lycopus europaeus	Radioactive iodine	May interfere, with administration of diagnostic procedures using radioactive isotopes
	Thyroid hormones	Should not be administered concurrently with preparations containing thyroid hormone.[11]
Uncaria tomentosa	HIV protease inhibitors	May increase drug level.
Capsicum spp.	Theophylline	May increase absorption antidrug level.
Apiumgraveolens	Thyroxine	May reduce serum levels of thyroxine.
Coleus forskohill	Antiplatelet Medication	May potentiate effects of drug
	Hypotensive medication	May potential effects of drug
	Prescribed medication	May potentiate effects of drug
	Prescribed medication	May potentiate effects of drug
Vaccinium macrocarpon	Midazolam	May increase drug levels
	Warfarin	May alter INR (most frequently increase)
Salvia miltiorrhiza	Midazolam	May decrease drug levels.
	Warfarin	May potentiate effect of drug.

TABLE 1 *Contd...*

Herbs	Drugs	Interaction
Harpagophytum procumbens	Warfarin	May increase bleeding tendency
Echinacea angustifolia	HIV protease egdarunavir	May decrease drug levels.
Echinacea angustifolia	Immunosuppressant medication	May decrease effectiveness of drug
	Midazolam	Decreases drug levels when drug administered intravenously
Denothera blennis	Phenothiazines	May decrease effectiveness of drug.
Allium sativum	Antiplatelet and antico-agulant drugs eg aspirin, warfarin	Aspirin: May increase bledding time.
		Warfarin: May potentiate effect of drug. Large doses could increase bleeding tendency.
	HIV protease inhibitors, e.g. saquina	Decreases drug level.
Zingiber officinale	Antacids	May decrease effectiveness of drug
	Antiplatelet and anticoagulant drugs e.g. phenprocoumon, warfarin	phenprpcoumon: May increase action of drug.
		Warfarin: Increased risk of spontaneous bleeding.
	Nifedipine	May produce a synergistic antiplatelet effect
Gingko biloba	Anticonvulsant medication, e.g. carbamazepine sodium, valproate.	May decrease. effectiveness of drug.
	Antiplatelet and anticoagulant drugs eg aspirin, clopidogrel, ticlopidine, warfarin	Prolongation of bleedingand /or increased bleeding tendency
	Antipsychotic medication eg haloperidol olanzapine, clozapine	May potentiate the efficiency of drug in patients with schizophrenia
	Benzodiazepines, eg. diazepam, midazolam	May alter drug level
	HIVnon-nucleoside transcriptase inhibitors egefavirenz	May decrease drug levels

TABLE 1 *Contd...*

Herbs	Drugs	Interaction
Gingko biloba	Hypoglycaemic drugs eg glipizide, metformin Pioglitazone, tolbutamide	Glipizide: May cause hypogly-caemia.
		Metformin: May enhance action of drug.
		Pioglitazone: May decrease effectiveness of drug
		Tolbutamide: May decrease effectiveness of drug
	Nifedipine	May increaswe drug levels or side effects.
	Omeprazole	May decrease drug levels.
	Talinolol	May increase drug levels
Hydrastis Canadensis	Drugs which displace the protein binding of billrubin e.g. phenybutazone	May potentiate effect of drug on displacing billrubin
	Midazolam	May increase drug level
Camallia sinensis	Boronic acid based protease inhibitors e.g. bortezomib	May decrease efficacy ofdrug.
	Folate	May decrease absorption
	Statin drugs eg simvastatin	May increase plasma level and side effect of drug.
	Warfarin	May inhibit effect of drug : decreased INR
Crataegus laevigata (c.owyacantha)	Digoxin	May increase effectiveness of drug
	Hypotensive drugs including betablockers	May increase effectiveness of drug
(Trigonella foenumgraecum) Gymmema sylvestre, Galega officinalis) Plantago ovata, p psylllium p Indica)	Hypolycaemic drugs, including Insulin	May potentiate hypoglycaemic activity of drug
Piper methysticum	CNS depressants, eg alcohol barbiturates benzodiazepines	Potentiation of drug effects
	L-Dopa and other Parkinson's disease treatments	Possible dopamine antagonist effects
Panax ginseng	Antihypertensive medications including nifedipine	Genera: May decrease effectiveness of drug

TABLE 1 *Contd...*

Herbs	Drugs	Interaction
Panax ginseng		Nifedipine: May increase drug levels
	Antiplatelet and anticoagulant drugs	General: May potentiate effects of drug.
		Warfarin: May decrease effectiveness of drug
	CNS stimulants	May potentiate effects of drug
	Hypoglycaemic drugs, including insulin	May potentiate hypoglycaemic activity of drug
	MAO inhibitors egphenelzine	Headache and tremor, mania
Laxative : **Aloe Barbadensis,** **Aloe ferox, Cassia** **spp, Rhamnus** **purshiana, Rumex** **crispus**	Antiarrhythmic agents	May affect activity if potassium deficiency resulting from long term lazative abuse is present
	Cardiac glycosides	May potentiate activity if potassium deficiency resulting from long-term laxative abuse is present
	Potassium depleting agents eg thiazide diuretics, corticosteroids, licorice not (glycylrrhiza Glabra)	May increase potassium depletion
Glycyrrhiza glabra	Antihypertensive medications other than diuretics	General: May decrease effectiveness of drug.
		ACE-inhibitor: May mask the development of Pseudoaldosteronism
	Cilostazol	May cause hypokalaemia, which can potentiate the toxicity of the drug.
	Digoxin	May cause hypokalaemia which can potentiate the toxicity of the drug.
	Diuretics	Spironolactone (potassium-sparing diuretic): reduced side effects of drug.
		Thiazide and loop (potassium depleting) diuretics: The combined effect of licorice and the drug could result in excessive potassium loss.

TABLE 1 *Contd...*

Herbs	Drugs	Interaction
Glycyrrhiza glabra	Immuno-supressives, egsirolimus	May decrease drug clearance.
	Midazolam	May decrease drug level
	Omeprazole	May decrease drug level
	Potassium depleting drugs other than thiazide and loop diuretics e.g. corticosteroids stimulant laxatives	The combined effect of licorice and the drug could result in excessive potassium loss
	Prednisolone	May potentiate the action or increase levels of drug
Athaea officinalis	Prescribed medication	May slow or reduce absorption of drugs
Fillpendula ulmaria	Warfrain	May potentiate effects of drug
Phellodendron amurense	Drugs that displace the protein binding of billrubin e.g. phenybutazone	May potentiate effect of drug on displacing billrubin
Capsicum annuum, Matricari-arecutita, Camellia sinensis, Tillacordata, Rosmarinus officinalis, Silyblurn-marianum, verbena officinalis	Iron	Inhibition of non-haem iron absorption
Plantago ovata, Plantago indica	Carbamazepine	Decreases plasma drug level
	Digoxin	May decrease absorption of drug
	Iron	Inhibition of non-haem iron absorption
	Lithium	May decrease absorption of drug
	Prescribed medication	May slow or reduce absorption of drugs
	Thyroxine	May decrease efficacy of drug
Schisandra Chinensis	Immunosupressives e.g. tacrolimus	May increase drug levels
Schisandra Chinensis	Midazolam	May increase drug levels
	Prescribed medication	May accelerate clearance from the body
	Talinolol	May increase drug levels possible effect on inhibiting p-gp
Eleutherococcus senticosun	Digoxin	May increase plasma drug levels
Ulmus rubra	Prescribed medication	May slow or reduce absorption of drugs

TABLE 1 *Contd...*

Herbs	Drugs	Interaction
Hypericum perforatum	Amitriplyline	Decrease drug levels
	Anticonvulsants e.g. carbamazepine, mephenytoin-phenobarbitone, phenytoin	May decrease drug levels via CYP induction
	Anthistamineeg fexofenadine	Decreases drug levels
	Antiplatelet and anticoagulant drugs egclopidogrel, phenprocoumon, warfarin	Clopidogrel: May potentiate effects of drugs
		Phenprocoumon: decreases plasma drug levels.
		Warfarin: decreases drug levels and INR
	Benzodiazepines, eg alprazolam, midazolam, quazepam	Decreases drug levels and is probably dependent upon the hyperforin content
	Calcium channel antagonists egnifedipine, verapamil	Decreases drug levels
	Cancer chemotherapeutic drugs eg irinotecan imatinib	Decreases drug levels
	Digoxin	Decreases drug levels
	Finasteride	May decrease drug levels
	HIV non-nucleoside transcriptase inhibitors egindinavir	Decreases drug levels
	Hypoglycaemic drugs e.g. gliclazlidetolbutamide	Gliclazide: May reduce efficacy ofdrug by increased clearance
Hypericum perforatum		Tolbutamide: May affect blood glucose
	Immuno suppressive e.g. cyclosporin, tacrollmus	Decreases drug levels
	Ivabradine	May decrease drug levels
	Methadone	Decrease drug levels possibly inducing withdrawal symptoms.
	Methylphenidate	May decrease efficacy
	Omeprazole	May decrease drug levels
	Oral contraceptives	May increase metabolism of drug
	Oxycodone	Decrease drug levels
	SSRls, e.g. paroxetine, trazodone, sertraline and other serotonergic agents eg. nefazodone, Venlafaxine	Potentiation effecs possible with regard to serotonin levels
	Statin drugs	May decrease effect and /or drug levels

TABLE 1 *Contd...*

Herbs	Drugs	Interaction
	Talinolol	May decrease drug levels
	Theophylline	May decrease drug levels
	Voriconazole	Decreases drug levels
	Zolpidem	May decrease drug levels (but with wide inter subject variability)
Silybum marianum	Hypoglycaemic drugs, including insulin	May improve insolin sensitivity
	Immuno suppressive segsirolimus	May decrease drug clearance
	Metronidazole	May decrease absorption rate of drug
	Omidazole	May increase drug levels
	Talinolol	May increase drug levels
Agrimonia eupatoria, Arctostaphylos uvaursh, Geranium maculatum, Vitis vinifera, Camellia sinensis, Crataegus app, Melissa officinalls, Filpendula ulmaria, Menthax piperita, Pelargonium sidoides, Pinusmas sonlana, Rubus idaeus, Salvia fruticosa, Hypericum perforatum, Salix spp.	Minerals especially iron	Iron: May reduce absorption of non haem iron from food Zinc: May reduce absorption for food. Clinical studies with healthy volunteers: results conflicting for effect on zinc (underfined tea, black tea consumed at or immediately after food.
Curcuma longa	Talinolol	May decrease drug levels
Valeriana eduilis, Valeriana officinalis	CNS depressants or alcohol	May potentiate effects of drug
Salix aiba, Salix daphnoides, Salix purpurea, Salix fragilis	Warfarin	May potentiate effect of drug.

PART - C
FOOD-DRUG INTERACTIONS

Numerous medicines have influential ingredients that interact with the human body in different ways. Diet and lifestyle can sometimes have a significant impact on drugs. A drug interaction is a situation in which a substance affects the activity of a drug, i.e. the effects are increased or decreased, or they produce a new effect that neither produces on its own. Typically, interactions between drugs come to mind (drug-drug interaction). However, interactions may also exist between drugs and foods (drug-food interactions), as well as drugs and herbs (drug-herb interactions).

These may occur out of accidental misuse or due to lack of knowledge about the active ingredients involved in the relevant substances. Interactions between food and drugs may inadvertently reduce or increase the drug effect. Some commonly used herbs, fruits as well as alcohol may cause failure of the therapy up a point of to serious alterations of the patient's health. The majority of clinically relevant food-drug interactions are caused by food-induced changes in the bioavailability of the drug.

Foremost side-effects of some diet (food) on drugs include alteration in absorption by fatty, high protein and fiber diets. Bioavailability is an important pharmacokinetic parameter which is correlated with the clinical effect of most drugs. However, in order to evaluate the clinical relevance of a food-drug interaction the impact of food intake on the clinical effect of the drug has to be quantified as well.

The majority important interactions are those coupled with a high risk of treatment failure arising from a significantly reduced bioavailability in the fed state. Such interactions are frequently caused by chelation with components in food. In addition, the physiological response to food intake, in particular, gastric acid secretion, may reduce or increase the bioavailability of certain drugs.

Drug interactions can alter the pharmacokinetics and/or pharmaco-dynamics of a drug. The pharmacodynamic interaction may be additive, synergistic, or antagonistic effects of a drug. Factors such as nonspecific binding, atypical kinetics, poor effector solubility, and varying ratios of accessory proteins may alter the kinetic behavior of an enzyme and subsequently confound the extrapolation of in vitro data to the human situation. Coenzyme Q-10 (CoQ10) is very widely consumed by humans as a food supplement because of its recognition by the public as an important nutrient in supporting human health. It interferes with intestinal efflux transporter P-glycoprotein (P-gp) and as result food-drug interactions arise.

The interaction of natural products and drugs is a common hidden problem encountered in clinical practice. The interactions between natural products and drugs are based on the same pharmacokinetic and pharmacodynamic principles as drug-drug interactions. Several fruits and berries have recently been shown to contain agents that affect drug-metabolizing enzymes. Grapefruit is the most well-known example, but also sevillian orange, pomelo and star fruit contain agents that inhibit cytochrome P450 3A4 (CYP3A4), which is the most important enzyme in drug metabolism.

Clinical pharmacist **Steve Plogsted**, educated us in on five foods that most commonly interact with medications.

Grapefruit Juice

Fruit juice like Grapefruit juice has the capability to interact with medications in various ways. One way is by increasing the absorption of certain drugs — as is the case with some, but not all, cholesterol-lowering statins. MedinePlus recommends avoiding grapefruit juice if you are taking statins.

The juice can also cause the body to metabolize drugs abnormally, ensuing in lower or higher than normal blood levels of the drug. Many medications are affected in this way, including antihistamines, blood pressure drugs, thyroid replacement drugs, birth control, stomach acid-blocking drugs, and the cough suppressant dextromethorphan. It's best to avoid or significantly reduce intake of grapefruit juice when taking these medications.

But why is grapefruit juice of concern and not other citrus juices? According to Plogsted, grapefruit juice contains a class of compounds called furanocoumarins, which act in the body to alter the characteristics of these medications. Orange juice and other citrus juices do not contain these compounds. There is some concern for Seville oranges and the pummelo, which are relatives of the grapefruit.

Green Leafy Vegetables

Blood-thinning drugs such as Coumadin® (warfarin) interfere with vitamin K-dependent clotting factors. Eating too much green leafy vegetables, which are high in vitamin K, can decrease the ability of blood-thinners to prevent clotting. But you don't have to give up greens altogether. Problems arise from significantly and suddenly increasing or decreasing intake, as it can alter the effectiveness of the medicine. So eat your greens in consistent amounts.

Natural Black Licorice (Glycyrrhiza)

According to Plogsted, glycyrrhiza — a natural ingredient used to make black licorice — can deplete the body of potassium while causing an increased retention of sodium. When the body is depleted of potassium, the activity of digoxin, a medication used to treat heart failure, can be greatly enhanced, resulting in the heart not beating properly.

Glycyrrhiza can also decrease the effectiveness of high blood pressure medicines. And people taking Coumadin® (warfarin) should beware that glycyrrhiza can break down the drug, resulting in an increase in the body's clotting mechanism.

Excessive amounts of natural licorice should be avoided when taking all of these medications. However, Plogsted notes that artificially-flavored black licorice doesn't contain glycyrrhiza and is not of concern.

Salt Substitutes

Consumers taking digoxin for heart failure or ACE inhibitors for high blood pressure should be careful with salt substitutes, which most often replace sodium with potassium. With an increased consumption of potassium, the effectiveness of digoxin can be decreased, resulting in heart failure. And those taking ACE inhibitors might see a significant increase in blood potassium levels, as these drugs are known to increase potassium.

"There is no real need to avoid salt substitutes, although care should be taken when using the product," say Plogsted. "If the consumer has decreased kidney function they should discuss the use of salt substitutes with their doctor."

Tyramine-Containing Foods

High blood levels of the amino acid tyramine can cause an increase in blood pressure. Several medications interfere with the breakdown of tyramine, including monoamine oxidase inhibitors (MAOIs) which treat depression, and drugs used to treat the symptoms of Parkinson's disease. Plogsted advises those taking these drugs to steer clear of tyramine-rich foods. The list is lengthy and includes, but is not limited to: chocolate, aged and mature cheeses, smoked and aged/fermented meats, hot dogs, some processed lunch meats, fermented soy products and draft beers (canned and bottled beers are OK).

When receiving a prescription for a new medication or taking a new over-the-counter drug, Plogsted advises consumers to always read drug warning labels and ask their physician and/or pharmacist about which foods or other drugs they should avoid or be concerned about taking.

TABLE 1

Food -Drug interactions (accelerate the absorption of drugs)

Drug	Mechanism	Conclusion
Griseofulvin	Drug is lipid soluble, enhanced absorption with high-fat foods	Take with high- fat foods.
Propranolol	Food may reduce first-pass extraction and metabolism.	Take with food.
Spironolactone	Delayed gastric emptying permits dissolution and absorption, bile may solubilize the drug.	Take with food.

TABLE 2

Food-Drug interactions (delay the absorption of drugs)

Drug	Mechanism	Conclusion
Acetaminophen	High pectin foods act as adsorbant and protectant.	Take on empty stomach, if not contraindicated.
Digoxin	High-fiber, high-pectin foods bind to the drug.	Take drug at the same time as food. Avoid taking with high-fiber foods.
Levodopa	Drug competes with amino acids for absorption transport.	Avoid taking drug with high— protein foods.
Glipizide	Mechanism unknown.	Affects blood glucose; more potent when taken half an hour before meals.
Quinidine	Possibly protein binding.	May take with food tg, prevent gastrointestinal upset.
	Competitive absorption.	Avoid taking with high- protein foods.

TABLE 2 *Contd...*

Drug	Mechanism	Conclusion
Sulfonamides	Mechanism unknown.	Taking with meals may prolong gastric emptying.
Tetracyclines	Binds with calcium ions or iron salts forming insoluble chelates.	Take one hour before or two hours after meals; do not take with milk.

TABLE 3

Potassium rich foods-drug interactions

Food	Drug	Mechanism	ADR
Potassium rich food	ACEIs (lisinopril, etc.,) ARBs (losartan, etc.,) Direct renin inhibitors (aliskeron) or potassium sparing diuretics (spiranolactone, etc.)	• Lowering of aldosterone levels * Increase potassium retention	Hyperkalemia
Potassium rich foods	Digoxin	Increases potassium levels	Reduction of theropeutic activity

TABLE 4

Some drug-food interactions (Special Precautions)

Drug	Effects and Precautions
Antibiotics Cephalosporins, Penicillin, Erythromycin, Sulfa drugs, Tetracycline	Take on an empty stomach to speed absorption of the drugs. Don't take with fruit juice or wine, which decreases the drug's effectiveness. Increase the risk of Vitamin B12 deficiency. Dairy products reduce the drug's effectiveness. Lowers Vitamin C absorption.
Anticonvulsants Dilantin, Phenobarbital	Increase the risk of anemia and nerve problems due to deficiency of folate and other B vitamins.
Antidepressants Fluoxetine Lithium Tricyclics	Reduce appetite and can lead to excessive weight loss A low-salt diet increases the risk of lithium toxicity; excessive salt reduces the drug's efficacy. Many foods, especially legumes, meat, fish and foods high in Vitamin C, reduce absorption of the drugs.
Antihypertensives, Heart Medications ACE inhibitors, Alpha blockers, Digitalis	Take on an empty stomach to improve the absorption of the drugs. Take with liquid or food to avoid excessive drop in blood pressure.

TABLE 4 *Contd...*

Drug	Effects and Precautions
Diuretics Potassium sparing diuretics	Avoid taking with milk and high fiber foods, which reduce absorption, increases potassium loss. Increase the risk of potassium deficiency. Unless a doctor advises otherwise, don't take diuretics with potassium supplements or salt substitutes, which can cause potassium overload.
Asthma Drugs Pseudoephedrine Theophylline	Avoid caffeine, which increases feelings of anxiety and nervousness. High protein diet reduces absorption. Caffeine increases the risk of drug toxicity.
Heartburn and Ulcer Medications Antacids, Cimetidine, Famotidine, Sucralfate	Interfere with the absorption of many minerals; for maximum benefit, take medication one hour after eating. Avoid high protein foods, caffeine and other items that increase stomach acidity.
Hormone Preparations Oral contraceptives Steroids Thyroid drugs	Salty foods increase fluid retention. Drugs reduce the absorption of folate, vitamin B6 and other nutrients; increase intake of foods high in these nutrients to avoid deficiencies. Salty foods increase fluid retention. Increase intake of foods high in calcium, vitamin K, potassium and protein to avoid deficiencies. Iodine-rich foods lower the drug's efficacy.
Laxatives Mineral Oils	Overuse can cause a deficiency of vitamins A, D, E, and K.
Painkillers Aspirin and stronger nonsteroidal antiinflammatory drugs Codeine	Always take with food to lower the risk of gastrointestinal irritation; avoid taking with alcohol, which increases the risk of bleeding. Frequent use of these drugs lowers the absorption of folate and vitamin C. Increase fiber and water intake to avoid constipation.
Sleeping Pills, Tranquilizers Benzodiazepines	Never take with alcohol. Caffeine increases anxiety and reduce drug's effectiveness.

TABLE 5

Protein rich foods- drug interactions

Food	Drug	Mechanism	ADR
Protein rich foods	BETA BLOCKERS Metoprolol Propronolol	Enhanced absorption of propranolol. Increases bioavailability.	Bradycardia, Hypotension, Broncho-constriction.
Protein rich foods	Carbidopa Levodopa Theophylline	Decreases concentration & efficacy.	Bradycardia, Hypotension, Broncho-constriction.

TABLE 6

Examples of drugs taken with caffien their mechanism and ADR

Drugs Taken with Caffeine	Mechanism	ADR
Oral contraceptives, Prednisone, Ciprofloxacin Cimetidine	Inhibits metabolism of caffeine. Increases effect of caffeine	Cardiac arrhythmia
Theophylline	Inhibition of theophylline metabolism. Increases serum concentration of theophylline.	Jitteriness, Insomnia, Cardiac arrhythmia
Bronchodilators	Changes activity of bronchodilators.	Excitability, nervousness, rapid heart beat

TABLE 7

Grape juice-Drug interactions

Drugs with Grape Juice	Mecahnism of Action	Adverse Drug Reactions
1. Statins: Simvastatin Lovastatin etc.	Furanocoumarins of grape-fruit juice inhibits the metabolism of statins.	Elevated risk of rhabdomyolysis.
2. Erythromycine Terfenadine Amiodarone Dronedarone Domperidone Nilotinib	FJ induces the prolongation of QT interval of heart beat by inhibiting the metabolism.	Increased risk of torsade de pointes
3. Calcium channel blockers: Felodipine Manidipine Nisoldipine	Inhibits the metabolism of calcium channel blockers.	Hypotension, Headache, flushing, oedema
4. Oral Contraceptives; Ethinylestradiol	Inhibits the metabolism of ethinylestradiol.	Elevated risk of deep vein thrombosis
5. Immuno-suppresants: Tacrolimus, Sirolimus Cyclosporine	GFJ inhibits the CYP3A4 mediated metabolism.	Elevated risk of nephrotoxicity
6. Opioids: Oxycodone, Fentanyl, Alfentanil	GFJ inhibits the CYP3A4 mediated metabolism.	Elevated risk of respiratory depression

TABLE 7 *Contd...*

Drugs with Gape Juice	Mecahnism of Action	Adverse Drug Reactions
7. Benzodiapezine: Diazepam, Midazolam Triazolam	Inhibits the metabolism of benzodiazepines.	Excessive sedation and amnesia
8. Selective Serotonin Reuptake Inhibitors (SSRIs): Fluoxetine, sertraline	Inhibits the metabolism of SSRIs.	Increased risk of serotonin syndrome

TABLE 8

Different fruit juices-Drug interactions

JUICE	DRUG	MOA	ADR
Apple juice (AJ)	Flexofenadine Cyclosporine Aliskiren	AJ inhibits OAPT (Organinc Anion Transport Polypeptide) and decreases the absorption of drug.	Diminished therapeutic efficacy.
Orange juice	Flexifebadine Aliskiren beta blockers (atenolol, Celeprolol, talindolol) Or fluoroquinolones (ciprofloxacin, Levofloxacine)	Decreases the absorption of drugs by inhibiting the OAPT (Organic Anion Transporting Polypeptide).	Reduction of therapeutic efficacy.
Pomelo orange	Felodipine, Cyclosporine or Tacrolimus	Pomelo orange inhibits the CYP3A4 mediated metabolism	Increased risk of adverse effects.
Seville orange	Dextrometharphen, Felodipine	Furanocoumarins of Seville orange juice inhibits CTP3A4 and decrease the metabolism.	Excessive adverse effects.

CHAPTER 3

Adverse Drug Reaction (ADR)

Adverse Drug Reaction can be defined as any unintended, undesirable or unexpected effect of a prescribed medication. According to WHO definition, any noxious, unintended, undesired effect of a drug which occurs at doses used for prophylaxis, diagnosis, or therapy, excluding therapeutic failures, intentional and accidental overdose and drug abuse, and does not include adverse effects due to errors in drug administration.

History behind the Adverse Drug Reaction Study

Van doeveren, professor of medicine provides early example of awareness of adverse drug effect when he gives the academic lecture called remedio amorbi in 1789 on dialysis caused by treatment. **Meyler**, in his famous book on adverse drug reaction in 1951 "side effect of drugs" focused attention on Van doeveren academic lecture. Systematic attention to adverse drug reaction, including the collection of adverse drug reaction reports, was boosted by the so-called thalidomide disaster in the early 1960s. In 1971 study by **Lely**, who discovered that 19 people died from digitalis intoxication caused by a production error of the digitalis tablets, was another eye opener. Following the thalidomide disaster in early 1960s, the World health Organization set up its international drug-monitoring programme. Since 1978 the programme is being carried out by the **Uppsala monitoring centre** (UMC) in Sweden, which is responsible for the collection of data about adverse reactions from around the world. UMC is engaged in editing, updating and publishing the drug dictionary. It is maintaining and publishing the adverse reaction Terminology (WHO-ART) and carrying out special searches of the database by request. The aim is not to ban any drug as banning a drug also depends on various factors like risk-benefit ratio. UMC is attempting to ensure that the ADRs are minimized and the positive effects of the drugs are enhanced through proper usage.

Historical landmark of Advese Drug Reaction

1880	.....	Chloroform - Cardiac arrest.
1922	.....	Organo-Arsenical compounds caused epidemic jaundice and fatal hepatic necrosis.
1946	.....	Streptomycin – deafness.
1954	.....	Blood dyscrasias with Chloramphenicol.
1961	.....	Thalidomide – phocomelia.
1970	.....	practolol causes oculomucocutaneous syndroms.
1975	.....	Clozapine – agranulocytosis.
1979	....	Triazolam – Psychosis.
1987	.....	Ofloxacin – Psychosis.
1998	.....	Sildenafil - stroke, myocardial infarction, cardiac arrest and hypertension.
1993-1999	.....	Nimuselide – national surveillance center for ADR reported acute fulminant hepatitis.
2000	.....	Cisapride – Prolonged the QT interval and cause Torsades De Pointes and ventricular tracycardia and death.
2002	....	Gatifloxacin induced prolongation of QTc interval leading dangerous arrhythmia, hypoglycemia.
2003	....	Roficoxib – cardiac arrhythmia.

Reason for Adverse Drug Reactions

- Over prescribing (Polypharmacy)
- Self medicatiom
- Prior history of ADRs
- Failure to setup a therapeutic end point by the physicians
- Difference in Bioavailibility of different brands
- Patient physiological factors like age, sex, diseased conditions like hepatitis or renal failure
- Genetic predisposition
- Drug interaction (enzyme inducting & inhibiting)

Why should we study Adverse Drug Reaction (ADR)?

We should study the ADR in order to understand the drug reaction in the following cases:

- Any drugs which are administered to patients can cause an ADR
- Peri operatively, multiple agents are administered which may lead to an adverse drug reaction.
- Fatal ADRs may cause death
- 30% of medical inpatients develop ADR
- 3% of all hospital admissions are due to ADRs
- Risk of an allergic reaction is approximately 1-3% for most administered drugs.

Severity of adverse drug reaction: On the basis of severity of ADR we can classify ADR under the following type:

Minor: In case of minor ADR no therapy is required, only antidote or prolongation of hospitalization is required.

Moderate: Patients with moderate ADR require changes in drug therapy, specific treatment or prolong hospital stay by atleast one day.

Severe: Severe ADR is potentially life threatening which may cause permanent damage or require intensive medical treatment.

Lethal: In case of lethal drug reaction, it directly or indirectly contributes to death of the patient

Classification of Adverse Effects

Adverse effects can be classified as Predictable and Unpredictable reactions.

Predictable (Type A or Augmented Reaction): This type of reaction is based on Pharmacological properties of the drug. Qualitatively normal response to the drug includes side effects, toxic effects and consequences of drug withdrawal.

Unpredictable (Type B or Bizarre Reaction): This type of effect is based on peculiarities of the patient and not on drug's known action; including allergy and idiosyncrasy. They are less common often requiring withdrawal of the drug.

TABLE 3.1

Adverse drug effects may be categorized into

Categorization	Definition	Examples
Side effects	These are unwanted but often unavoidable Pharmacodynamic effects that occur at therapeutic dose.	Atropin used show anti secretary action
Secondary effects	These are indirect consequences of a primary action of the drug.	Suppression of bacterial flora by tetracyclines paves the way for super infections.
Intolerance	It is the appearance of characteristic toxic effects of drug in an individual at therapeutic dose.	Single dose of Triflupromazine cause muscular dystonias in some individual. Specially in children
Idiosyncrasy	It is the abnormal reactivity to a chemical. The drug interacts with some unique feature of individual, not found in majority of subjects and produces the uncharacteristic reaction.	Barbituratus cause excitement & mental confusions in some individuals.
Drug allergy	It is an immunologicaliy mediated reaction producing stereotype symptoms which are unrelated to the Pharmaco-dynamic profile of the drug	Itching, Aplastic Anemia, Rashes, Contact Dermatitis.
Photosensitivity	It is a cutaneous reaction resulting from drug induced sensitization of the skin to UV radiation.	Local Tissue damage (Sun burn), like Erythema, Edema.
Drug dependence	It is a state in which use of drug for personal satisfaction is accorded a higher priority than other basic needs, often risks the health.	Amphetamines produce little or no physical dependences.
Withdrawal Reaction	Apart from drugs that are usually recognised as producing dependence, sudden interruption of therapy with certain other drugs also results in adverse consequence, mostly in the form of worsening of the clinical condition for which the drug was being used.	Severe hypertension, restlessness and sympathetic over activity may occur after discontinuation of Clonidine.
Teratogenicity	It refers to capacity of a drug to cause foetal abnormalities when administrated to pregnant women.	Thalidomide disaster

Definitions

Harm: Impairment of the physical, emotional, or psychological function of structure of the body and/or pain resulting there from.

Monitoring: To observe or record relevant physiological or psychological change.

Intervention: May include change in therapy or active medical/surgical treatment.

Intervention necessary to sustain life: Includes cardiovascular and respiratory support (e.g., CPR, defibrillation, intubation etc.)

National Coordinating Council (NCC) MERP Index for Categorizing Medication Errors

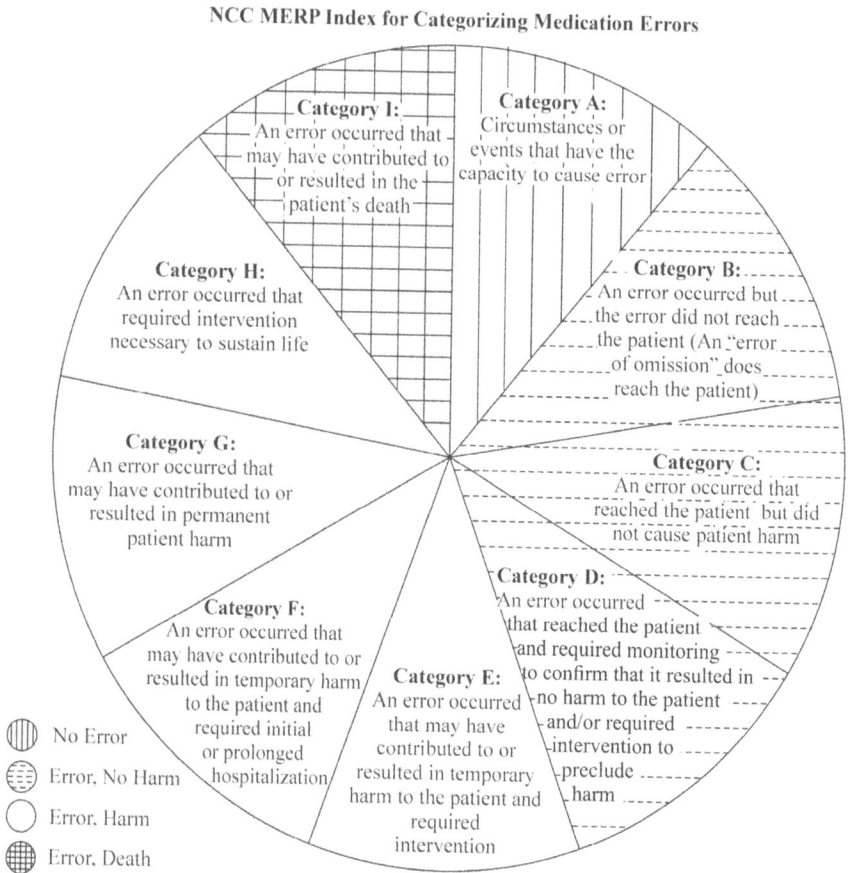

NCC MERP Index for Categorizing Medication Errors

Category I: An error occurred that may have contributed to or resulted in the patient's death

Category A: Circumstances or events that have the capacity to cause error

Category H: An error occurred that required intervention necessary to sustain life

Category B: An error occurred but the error did not reach the patient (An "error of omission" does reach the patient)

Category G: An error occurred that may have contributed to or resulted in permanent patient harm

Category C: An error occurred that reached the patient but did not cause patient harm

Category F: An error occurred that may have contributed to or resulted in temporary harm to the patient and required initial or prolonged hospitalization

Category E: An error occurred that may have contributed to or resulted in temporary harm to the patient and required intervention

Category D: An error occurred that reached the patient and required monitoring to confirm that it resulted in no harm to the patient and/or required intervention to preclude harm

No Error
Error, No Harm
Error, Harm
Error, Death

Definitions
Harm: Impairment of the physical, emotional, or psychological function or structure of the body and/or pain resulting therefrom.
Monitoring: To observe or record relevant psychological or psychological signs.
Intervention: May include change in therapy or active medical/surgical treatment.
Intervention necessary to sustain life Includes cardiovascular and respiratory support (eg, CPR, defibrillation, intubation, etc.)

Fig. 3.1

TABLE 3.2

List of Drugs with ADR

Name of Drugs	Adverse Drug Reactions (ADR)
Acebutolol (Adrenergic)	Constipation; diarrhea; dizziness or lightheadedness; frequent urination; gas; headache; indigestion; mild drowsiness; nausea; sleepiness unusual tiredness or weakness.
Acetaminophen (Analgesic & antipyretic)	Nausea, upper stomach pain, itching, loss of appetite and jaundice.
Acetohexamide (Anti diabetic)	Swelling, rapid weight gain, increased urination, pale or yellowed skin, dark coloured urine, fever and confusion,
Acetylprocainamide (Local anaesthetic)	Headache, dizziness, fatigue; cough; somnolence, nausea and hypotension.
Acetyl Salicylic acid (Antipyretic-analgesic)	Ringing in your ears, confusion, hallucinations, rapid breathing, seizure (convulsions) and severe nausea.
Acetylcysteine (Respiratory agent)	Wheezing, tightness in chest, difficulty in breathing, Skin rash or other irritation, Clammy skin, fever,
Acrosoxacin (Quinolone antibiotic)	Nausea, vomiting, heartburn, constipation, diarrhoea, abdominal cramping, anorexia; headache and dizziness.
Acetazolamide (Antiepileptic)	Confusion, Convulsions, Drowsiness, Flaccid, paralysis, Malaise, Paresthesias, Photosensitivity, Urticaria, Anorexia, Diarrhea and Metallic taste.
Actinomycin (Antiviral)	Black, tarry stools, blood in the urine or stools, cough or hoarseness accompanied by fever or chills, diarrhea (continuing), difficulty with swallowing, fever or chills and heartburn.
Acyclovir (Antiviral)	Lethargy, tremors, confusion, and seizures, pain, swelling, Abdominal or stomach pain, decreased frequency of urination and amount of urine.
Adrenaline (Sympathomimetis)	Severe low blood pressure, wheezing, severe skin itching, hives, and other symptoms of an allergic reaction.
Ajmaline (Antiarrythmic)	Heart block; cardiac arrhythmias; eye twitching; convulsions; respiratory depression; hepatotoxicity and agranulocytosis.
Albendazole (Anthelmintics)	Hypersensitivity-reactions, including rash andurticaria, granulocytopenia, pancytopenia and agranulocytosis.
Aldesleukin (Interleukin)	Fever and chills or flu-like symptoms,Generalized flushing (redness) of the face and body, or skin rash, Nausea or vomiting, Lowered blood pressure, Diarrhea and Low blood count.

TABLE 3.2 Contd...

Name of Drugs	Adverse Drug Reactions (ADR)
Alfentanil (Opioid analgesic)	Nausea, vomiting, heartburn, constipation, diarrhoea, abdominal cramping, anorexia; headache and dizziness.
Allopurinol (Antigout)	Ankle, knee, or great toe joint pain, joint stiffness or swelling, rash and rash with flat lesions or small raised lesions on the skin.
Alphaxalone (Antiaesthetic)	Depression apnoea and hypoxia, increased or decreased heart rate, and increased or decreased blood pressure.
Amlodipine (Antihypertensive)	Swelling of the ankles or feet, Difficult or laboured breathing, dizziness, fast, irregular, pounding, or racing heartbeat or pulse, feeling of warmth, redness of the face, neck, arms, and occasionally, upper chest and shortness of breath.
Aminocaproic acid (Antifibrinolytic)	Weakness, especially on one side of the body; sudden headache, confusion, problems with vision, nausea, vomiting, stomach pain or cramping, diarrhea, headache, dizziness, hallucinations (seeing things or hearing voices that do not exist), swelling of the arms, hands, feet, ankles, or lower legs and ringing in the ear.
Aminopyrine (Analgesic)	Fever, asthenia, fatigue, arrhythmia, palpitation, cholestatic jaundice, hepatitis, liver enzyme abnormalities, Changes in menstrual periods, decreased sexual ability in male, dry, puffy skinswelling of front part of neck and weight gain (unusual).
Aminosalicylic acid (Antimycobacterial)	Fever, skin, dermatitis, syndrome, leucopenia, agranulo-cytosis, hemolytic anemia, joint pains skin rash or itching and unusual tiredness or weakness.
Amitriptyline (Antidepressant)	Myocardial infarction; stroke; nonspecific ECG changes and changes in AV conduction; heart block, Abdominal or stomach pain, blood in urine or stools, blurred vision continuing ringing, buzzing, or other unexplained noise in ears, convulsions, cool and pale skin cough or hoarseness.
Amodiaquine (Antimalarial)	Dizziness or vertigo; acute renal failure, interstitial nephritis, acute tubular necrosis and electrolyte imbalances.
Amoxycillin (Antibiotic)	Headache, nausea, dizziness, vomiting, diarrhoea, black hairy tongue, maculopapular rash, urticaria, eosinophilia, Skin rash, itching or hives, swelling of the face, lips.
Amphetamine (CNS Stimulant)	Bladder pain bloody or cloudy urine, difficult, burning, or painful urinationfast, pounding, or irregular heartbeat or pulse, frequent urge to urinate and lower back or side pain.
Amphotericin (Antifungal)	Topical: Local irritation, pruritus and skin rash. IV infusion: Fever, chills, convulsions, malaise; nausea, vomiting, fever (sometimes accompanied by shaking chills usually occurring within 15 to 20 minutes after initiation of treatment); malaiseand weight loss.

TABLE 3.2 *Contd...*

Name of Drugs	Adverse Drug Reactions (ADR)
Ampicillin (Antibiotic)	GI upset, nausea, vomiting, diarrhoea; blood dyscrasias; urticaria, exfoliative dermatitis, rash and fever.
Amrinone (Inotropic agent)	GI disturbances, nausea, vomiting, thrombocytopaenia, hypotension, chest pain, hypersensitivity, Vomiting, and Abdominal pain.
Amsacrine (Antineoplastic)	Fatigue (tiredness), sore mouth and throat, loss of fertility, absence of menstrual period, and decrease in the number of healthy white blood cells, red blood cells.
Amylobarbitone (Sedative)	Hypersensitivity, dizziness, diarrhoea, nausea, vomiting, renal impairment, rash, erythema multiforme.
Anistreplase (Thrombolytic drug)	Allergic reactions; fever; nausea and vomiting; haemorrhage; hypotension and pulmonary embolism.
Antipyrine (Analgesic)	GI disturbances, nausea, diarrhoea, rash, bruising, Severe allergic reactions (rash; hives; itching; difficulty breathing; tightness in the chest; swelling of the mouth, face, lips, or tongue); irritation not present when you began using antipyrine/benzocaine.
Apomorphine (Antispycotic)	Nausea and vomiting; dyskinesia; dizziness; yawning; drowsiness; transient sedation and postural hypotension.
Aspirin (Analgesic & antipyretic)	GI disturbances, epigastric discomfort, prolonged bleeding time, rhinitis, urticaria; angioedema, salicylism, Vomiting, Stomach pain, Heartburn, Drowsiness and Nausea.
Astemazole (Antihistamin)	GI upset, glossitis, stomatitis and altered taste
Atenolol (Antihypertensive)	Bronchospasm; cold extremities, fatigue, dizziness, insomnia, lethargy, confusion, headache, depression, slow or uneven heartbeats and feeling light-headed, fainting; feeling short of breath, even with mild exertion.
Atracurium (Neuromuscular blocker)	Cutaneous reactions; bradycardia, transient hypotension in patients with CVS disorders; dyspnoea and bronchospasm.
Atropine (Analgesic & antipyretic)	Dry mouth, dysphagia, constipation, flushing and dryness of skin, tachycardia, palpitations, arrhythmias, mydriasis, ventricular fibrillation, supraventricular or ventricular tachycardia, dizziness, nausea, blurred vision, loss of balance, dilated pupils, photophobia, dry mouth and potentially extreme confusion, dissociative hallucinations and excitation especially amongst the elderly.
Auranofin (Antiimflarnmatory)	GI disturbances (nausea, vomiting, abdominal pain, diarrhoea, pruritus, rash; dermatitis, itching or skin rash, white patches or sores inside your mouth or on your lips, pain or swelling in your gums or tongue, metallic taste in your mouth, severe or ongoing diarrhea, severe nausea, vomiting, stomach cramps.

TABLE 3.2 *Contd...*

Name of Drugs	Adverse Drug Reactions (ADR)
Aurothiomalate (Anti gout)	Skin and mucous membrane reactions; stomatitis with a metallic taste; rash with pruritus and GI disorders.
Azapropazone (Antiinflammatory)	GI disorders; hypersensitivity reactions, headache, dizziness, nervousness, depression anddrowsiness,
Azathioprine (Immunosup-pressant)	Fever, chills; bone marrow depression characterised by leucopenia, thrombocytopenia or anaemia and anorexia.
Azelastin (Tropical Nasopharyngal Medication)	Irritation, stinging and itching of the nasal mucosa. Sneezing, nosebleeds, headache; nausea and taste disturbances.
Azlocillin (Antibiotic)	Pain at the injection site and phlebitis; electrolyte disturbances and dose-dependent coagulation defect.
Aztreonam (Antibacterial)	Phloebitis and thrombophloebitis. IM: Pain and swelling at injection site; diarrhoea, nausea, vomiting and altered taste.
Azithromycin (Antibacterial)	Mild to moderate nausea, vomiting, abdominal pain, dyspepsia, flatulence, diarrhoea, cramping and angioedema.
Bacampicillin (Antibiotic)	Hypersensitivity reactions including uticaria; fever; joint pains; rashes and angioedema.
Bacitracin (Antibacterial)	Nausea, vomiting, hypersensitivity reactions, Nephrotoxic reactions, Albuminuria and cylindruria.
Baclofen (Muscle Relaxant)	Sedation, drowsiness, ataxia, dizziness, headache, confusion, hallucinations, skin reactions, GI symptoms. Headache, insomnia, euphoria, excitement, and depression.
Bacmecillinam (Antibiotic)	Hypersensitivity reactions including angioedema, urticariaa and rash.
Bamethan (Calcium antagonist)	Headache, dizziness, back pain, myalgia, respiratory tract disorders, asthenia/fatigue, and first dose hypotension and rash.
Barbital (Hypnotic)	Dizziness, clumsiness, sleepiness, staggering walk, drowsiness, vomiting, tiredness, nausea and loss of appetite, headache, nightmares and constipation.
Beclomethasone (Cortico Steroid)	Loss of skin collagen and SC atrophy; local hypopigmentation of deeply pigmented skin; dryness, hypersensitivity reactions, urticaria, angioedema, rash, and bronchospasm, aggression, depression and sleep disorders.
Benazepril (Anti hypertensive)	Chills, cold sweats, confusion, dizziness, faintness, or lightheadedness when getting up suddenly from a lying or sitting position, unusual tiredness or weakness, Arm, back, or jaw pain, blistering, peeling, or loosening of the skin, bloating or swelling of the face.
Bendrofluazide (Cardiovascular agent)	Feeling faint when standing up, Feeling sick (nausea), Vomiting, Diarrhoea and Constipation.

TABLE 3.2 *Contd...*

Name of Drugs	Adverse Drug Reactions (ADR)
Benorylate (Analgesic)	Heartburn, GI disturbances, drowsiness and hypersensitivity reactions. Occasionally dizziness, tinnitus, deafness, nausea, constipation, indigestion, heartburn, drowsiness, dizziness and skin rashes.
Benoxaprofen (Anti inflammatory)	Dizziness or vertigo; acute renal failure, interstitial nephritis, acute tubular necrosis; electrolyte imbalances, photosensitivity, onycholysis, rash, milia, increased nail growth, pruritus and hypertrichosis.
Benperidol (Anti psychotic)	Dizziness or vertigo; acute renal failure, interstitial nephritis, acute tubular necrosis; electrolyte imbalances. Tardive dyskinesia, Drowsiness, Extrapyramidal reactions, Parkinsonism, Akathisia and Impairment of alertness.
Benzafibrate (Lipid lowering agent)	GI upset; pruritus, urticaria, alopoecia, impotence; vertigo, fatigue; nausea, vomiting, itching, hives, muscle pain, dizziness, hair loss, impotence, fainting, fatigue and increase in liver enzymes.
Benzylpenicillin (Antibiotic)	Hypersensitivity reactions including uticaria; fever; joint pains; rashes and angioedema.
Bepridil (Calcium channel blocker)	Swelling of your lips, tongue, or face; or hives); fainting or severe dizziness; chest pain; abnormal behavior or psychosis; yellowing of your skin or eyes (jaundice); or swelling of your legs or ankles, unusual fatigue or tiredness; nausea, upset stomach, diarrhea, or constipation; headache; nervousness or mild dizziness and insomnia.
Betahistine (Antileutic)	Headaches, indigestion, nausea, anaphylactic reactions, angioedema, gastrointestinal problems such as stomach pain or distension, vomiting, hypersensitivity reactions, itching, skin rash or rashes and urticaria.
Betamethasone (Corticosteroid)	Sodium and fluid retention, potassium and calcium depletion. Muscle wasting, weakness, osteoporosis. Intra-articular and soft-tissue injection: Soft-tissue atrophy, hypopigmentation or hyperpigmentation, facial erythema, thin, fragile skin.
Betaxolol (Drug for Glucoma)	Chest pain or discomfort, lightheadedness, dizziness, or fainting, shortness of breath, slow or irregular heartbeat, unusual tiredness, Cold arms, legs, hands, or feed, difficult or labored breathing, fast, pounding, or racing heartbeat or pulse, swelling of face, fingers, feet, or lower legs, tightness in the chest and wheezing.
Bethanidine (Antihypertensive)	Anxiety, tachycardia, tremor and dry mouth.

TABLE 3.2 Contd...

Name of Drugs	Adverse Drug Reactions (ADR)
Bevantolol (β-blocker and calcium channel blocker)	Bradycardia; hypotension; heart failure, heart block; bronchospasm; fatigue; coldness of extremities; pneumonitis. Anxiety, blurred vision, chills and cold sweats.
Bishydroxycoumarin (Anticoagulant)	Depressant, Hair loss, Nausea and vomiting, Mouth sores, Diarrhea, Skin problems, follicular acne and redness.
Bupivacaine (Local Anesthetic)	Hypotension, arrhythmia, bradycardia, heart block, cardiac arrest, vertigo, tinnitus, restlessness, anxiety, dizziness and seizure.
Buprenorphme (Analgesic & antipyretic)	Headache, Insomnia, Asthenia, Somnolence, Nausea, Dizziness, Sweating, Sedation, nausea, dizziness, vertigo, hypotension, miosis, headache, hypoventilation, respiratory or CNS depression.
Bupropion (Anti-depressant, smoking cessation drug)	Facial odema; nausea, dry mouth, constipation, diarrhoea, anorexia; mouth ulcer; thirst; myalgia, arthralgia. Postural hypotensionVasodilation, Syncope, Hypotension, Palpitations, Hallucinations, Irritability, Hostility and Seizures.
Burimamide (Anti ulcer Drug)	Headache, tiredness, dizziness, confusion, diarrhea, constipation and rash.
Buserelin (Hormone)	Depression or worsening of depression, mood changes, changes in level of lipids in the blood, headaches including migraines, hearing problemsand tinnitus.
Busulphan (Antineoplastic)	Interstitial pulmonary fibrosis, hyperpigmentation, seizures, hepatic, emesis, and wasting syndrome.
Butobarbitone (Sedative)	Drowsiness, ataxia, paradoxical excitement, confusion, headache and CNS depression and respiratory depression.
Butriptyline (Antidepressant)	Nausea, sweating, tremor, hypersensitivity reactions, behavioral, Hypersensitivity, dizziness and diarrhea.
Cadralazine (Anti hypertensive)	Arm, back, or jaw pain, chest pain or discomfort, chest tightness or heaviness, fast, pounding, or irregular heartbeat or pulse, nausea, shortness of breath and sweating.
Caffeine (CNS stimulant)	Diarrhea, dizziness, fast heartbeat, hyperglycemia, irritability, nervousness, or severe jitters (in newborn babies), nausea (severe), tremors and trouble in sleeping and Vomiting.
Capreomycin (Antitubercular)	Greatly increased or decreased frequency of urination or amount of urine, increased thirst, loss of appetite, nausea and vomiting.
Captopril (Anti hypertensive)	Cough, bradykinin, angioedema, agranulocytosis, proteinuria, hyperkalemia, taste alteration, teratogenicity, postural hypotension, acute renal failure and leucopenia.

TABLE 3.2 Contd...

Name of Drugs	Adverse Drug Reactions (ADR)
Carbamazepine (Anticonvulsant)	Drowsiness, dizziness, headaches and migraines, motor coordination impairment, nausea, vomiting, and/or constipation.
Carbimazole (Antithyroid)	Whilst rashes, pruritus, bone marrow, suppression causing neutropenia and agranulocytosis.
Carbenicillin (Antibacterial)	GI effects, including dose-related nausea, vomiting, diarrhea, abdominal cramps, and flatulence. Unpleasant after taste and smell.
Carbenoxolone (Antiulcer)	Sodium and water retention, hypokalaemia. Drug Interactions and Antagonism with amiloride.
Carbocysteine (Respiratory agent)	Allergic reactions, anaphylactic reactions, certain types of dermatitis, erythema multiforme, gastrointestinal bleeding, skin rash or rashes and Steven-Johnson syndrome.
Carboplatin (Antineoplastic)	Constipation; diarrhea; hair loss; loss of appetite; nausea; stomach pain or upset; vomiting and weakness.
Carisoprodol (Muscle Relaxant)	Paralysis (loss of feeling), extreme weakness or lack of coordination, feeling light-headed, fainting, fast heartbeat, seizure (convulsions), vision loss, agitation and confusion.
Carmustine (Antineoplastic)	Blurred vision, change in ability to see colors, especially blue or yellow, confusion, fever, headache, nausea and vomiting, problems with movement, walking, or speech, seizures and trouble healing.
Carprofen (Antiinflammatory)	Loss of appetite, Vomiting, Diarrhea, Increase in thirst, Increase in urination, Fatigue and/or Lethargy, Loss of coordination and Seizures.
Carvedilol (Antihypertensive)	Allergy, chest pain, discomfort, tightness, or heaviness, dizziness, lightheadedness, or fainting, generalized swelling or swelling of the feet, ankles, or lower legs, pain, shortness of breath, slow heartbeat and weight gain.
Cefacetrile (Antibiotic)	Diarrhea, Abdominal or stomach pain, blistering, peeling, or loosening of the skin, chills, clay-coloured stools and cough.
Cefaclor (Antibacterial)	Stomach upset, headache, nausea, vomiting, or diarrhea may occur.
Cefadroxil (Antibacterial)	Black, tarry stools, bleeding gums, blistering, peeling, or loosening of the skin, blood in the urine or stools, chills, clay-coloured stools, cough or hoarseness and dark-coloured urine and diarrhea.
Cephamandole (Broad spectrum antibiotic)	Gastrointestinal - Nausea and vomiting, Hypersensitivity - Rash, hives, eosinophilia, and drug fever and Severe - Kidney damage.

TABLE 3.2 Contd...

Name of Drugs	Adverse Drug Reactions (ADR)
Cefapirin (Antibacterial)	Nausea; vomiting; diarrhoea; hypersensitivity reactions; nephrotoxicity; convulsions and CNS toxicity.
Cefathiamidine (Antibacterial)	Dizziness or vertigo; acute renal failure, interstitial nephritis, acute tubular necrosis and electrolyte imbalances.
Cefatrizine (Antibacterial)	Nausea; vomiting; diarrhoea; hypersensitivity reactions; nephrotoxicity; convulsions; CNS toxicity; pseudomembranous colitis; hepatic dysfunction; haematologic disorders; pain at Injection site (IM); thrombophloebitis (IV infusion) and superinfection with prolonged use.
Cefazaflur (Antibacterial)	Nausea, vomiting, diarrhoea, abdominal discomfort; skin rash, angioedema; elevated liver enzyme values.
Cefazodone (Antidepressants)	Nausea, dry mouth, insomnia, somnolence, agitation, constipation, asthenia, dizziness, lightheadedness, orthostatic hypotension, confusion, blurred vision, abnormal vision, eye pain, sinus bradycardia, dyspnoea, bronchitis, syndrome of inappropriate secretion of anti-diuretic hormone and impotence.
Cefazolin (Antibacterial)	Diarrhoea, oral candidiasis, vomiting, nausea, stomach cramps, anorexia; eosinophilia, itching, drug fever, skin rash, Steven-Johnsons syndrome; neutropenia, leucopenia and thrombocytopenia,
Cefbuperazone (Antibacterial)	Skin rash, urticaria; eosinophilia, diarrhoea, nausea, vomiting; phloebitis; hypoprothrombinaemia and superinfection.
Cefixime (Antibacterial)	Diarrhoea, nausea, vomiting, abdominal pain; headache, dizziness, thrombocytopenia and eosinophilia.
Cefmenoxime (Antibacterial)	Nausea; vomiting; diarrhoea; hypersensitivity reactions; nephrotoxicity; convulsions; CNS toxicity; hepatic dysfunction; haematologic disorders; pain at Injection site (IM); thrombophloebitis (IV infusion) and superinfection with prolonged use.
Cefmetazole (Antibacterial)	Hypersensitivity reactions; nephrotoxicity; neutropenia; thrombocytopenia; agranulocytosis; bleeding complications related to hypoprothrombinaemia or platelet dysfunction; GI effects; CNS toxicity; superinfection; pain at Injection site (IM); thrombophloebitis (IV infusion); hepatitis and cholestatic jaundice.
Cefonicid (Antibacterial)	Dizziness or vertigo; acute renal failure, interstitial nephritis, acute tubular necrosis and electrolyte imbalances
Cefoperazone (Antibacterial)	Skin rash, urticaria; eosinophilia, diarrhoea, nausea, vomiting; phloebitis; hypoprothrombinaemia and superinfection.

TABLE 3.2 *Contd...*

Name of Drugs	Adverse Drug Reactions (ADR)
Ceforanide (Antibacterial)	Dizziness or vertigo; acute renal failure, interstitial nephritis, acute tubular necrosis and electrolyte imbalances.
Cefotaxime (Antibacterial)	Pain at Injection site; hypersensitivity reactions, rash, pruritus; diarrhoea, nausea, vomiting; candidiasis; eosinophilia, neutropenia, leucopenia and thrombocytopenia.
Cefotetan (Antibacterial)	Stomatitis, pharyngitis, dyspnoea and neuropathy.
Cefotiam (Second generation cephalosporin antibiotic)	Nausea; vomiting; diarrhoea; hypersensitivity reactions; nephrotoxicity; convulsions; CNS toxicity; hepatic dysfunction; haematologic disorders; pain at Injection site (IM); thrombophloebitis (IV infusion) and superinfection with prolonged use.
Cefoxitin (Antibacterial)	Nausea; vomiting; diarrhoea; hypersensitivity reactions; nephrotoxicity; convulsions; CNS toxicity; hepatic dysfunction; haematologic disorders; pain at Injection site (IM); thrombophloebitis (IV infusion); superinfection with prolonged use and Headache.
Cefpimizole (Antibacterial)	Dizziness or vertigo; acute renal failure, interstitial nephritis, acute tubular necrosis and electrolyte imbalances;
Cefpivamide (Antibacterial)	Hypersensitivity reactions including uticaria; fever; joint pains; rashes; angioedema; serum sickness-like reactions; haemolytic anaemia; interstitial nephritis; neutropaenia; thrombocytopaenia; CNS toxicity including convulsions; diarrhoea; nausea and vomiting.
Cefpodoxime (Antibacterial)	Anaphylactic shock; purpuric nephritis, skin rash, pruritus; diarrhoea, nausea, abdominal pain and vomiting.
Cefprozil (Antibacterial)	Nausea; vomiting; diarrhoea; hypersensitivity reactions; nephrotoxicity; convulsions; CNS toxicity; hepatic dysfunction; haematologic disorders; pain at Injection site (IM); thrombophloebitis (IV infusion) and superinfection with prolonged use.
Cefroxadmec (Antibacterial)	Nausea vomiting; diarrhea and hypersensitivity reactions;
Cefsulodin (Antibacterial)	Nausea; vomiting; diarrhoea; hypersensitivity reactions; nephrotoxicity; convulsions; CNS toxicity; hepatic dysfunction; haematologic disorders; pain at Injection site (IM); thrombophloebitis (IV infusion) and superinfection with prolonged use.
Cefsumide (Antibacterial)	Skin rash, urticaria; eosinophilia, diarrhoea, nausea, vomiting; phloebitis; hypoprothrombinaemia and superinfection

TABLE 3.2 *Contd...*

Name of Drugs	Adverse Drug Reactions (ADR)
Ceftazidime (Antibacterial)	Hypersensitivity, dizziness, diarrhoea, nausea, vomiting, renal impairment, rash, erythema multiforme, thrombocytopaenia, superinfection, phloebitis and thrombophloebitis at the site of injection.
Ceftezole (Antibacterial)	Nausea; vomiting; diarrhea; hypersensitivity reactions; nephrotoxicity; convulsions; CNS toxicity; hepatic dysfunction; hematologic disorders; pain at injection site (IM); thrombophlebitis (IV infusion); superinfection with prolonged use.
Ceftizoxime (Antibacterial)	Burning; rash, pruritus, fever; anorexia, nausea, vomiting, diarrhoea; rarely neutropaenia, leucopaenia, thrombocytopaenia. Transient elevations of transaminases (SGOT and SGPT) and alkaline phosphatase, transient rise in BUN and creatinine.
Ceftriaxone (Antibacterial)	Diarrhoea, nausea, vomiting; neutropenia, eosinophilia, anaemia, rash, pruritus, fever, chills, increased serum concentrations of AST, ALT, BUN; local reactions (e.g. pain, induration, ecchymosis, tenderness at Injection site). Rarely, pancreatitis and hypoprothrombinaemia.
Cefuroxime (Antibacterial)	Large doses can cause cerebral irritation and convulsions; nausea, vomiting, diarrhoea, GI disturbances; erythema multiforme, Stevens-Johnson syndrome and epidermal necrolysis.
Celiprolol (Anti hypertensive)	Headache, fatigue, dizziness, hot flushes, asthenia, somnolence and insomnia; tremor and palpitations; bronchospasm, skin rashes and/or visual disturbances. Rarely, depression and hypersensitivity pneumonitis.
Cephalexin (Antibiotic)	GI disturbances (e.g. nausea, vomiting, diarrhoea, abdominal discomfort), dyspepsia; allergic reactions (e.g. rash urticaria, angioedema); genital and anal pruritus, genital candidiasis, vaginitis and vaginal discharge, dizziness, fatigue, headache, agitation, confusion, hallucinations and arthralgia
Cephalexm (Antibacterial)	GI disturbances (e.g. nausea, vomiting, diarrhoea, abdominal discomfort), dyspepsia; allergic reactions (e.g. rash urticaria, angioedema); genital and anal pruritus, genital candidiasis, vaginitis and vaginal discharge, dizziness, fatigue, headache and agitation.
Cephaloglycin (Antibiotic)	Vomiting; diarrhoea; hypersensitivity reactions; nephrotoxicity; convulsions; CNS toxicity and pseudomembranous.
Cephaloridine (Antibacterial)	Neurotoxicity, ototoxicity, nephrotoxicity and skin rash.

TABLE 3.2 Contd...

Name of Drugs	Adverse Drug Reactions (ADR)
Cephalothin (Antibacterial)	Nausea; vomiting; diarrhoea; hypersensitivity reactions; nephrotoxicity; convulsions; CNS toxicity; pseudo-membranous colitis; hepatic dysfunction; haematologic disorders; pain at Inj site (IM); thrombophloebitis (IV infusion); superinfection with prolonged use.
Cepnamandole (Antibacterial)	Nausea; vomiting; diarrhoea; hypersensitivity reactions; nephrotoxicity; convulsions; CNS toxicity; pseudo-membranous colitis; hepatic dysfunction; haematologic disorders; pain at inj site (IM); thrombophloebitis (IV infusion); superinfection with prolonged use.
Cephaprim (Antibacterial)	Nausea; vomiting; diarrhoea; hypersensitivity reactions; nephrotoxicity; convulsions and CNS toxicity.
Cephazolin (Antibacterial)	Diarrhoea, oral candidiasis, vomiting, nausea, stomach cramps, anorexia; eosinophilia, itching, drug fever, skin rash, Stevens-Johnson syndrome; neutropenia, leucopenia and thrombocytopenia.
Cephradame (Antibacterial)	Dizziness or vertigo; acute renal failure, interstitial nephritis, acute tubular necrosis; electrolyte imbalances.
Chloral hydrate (Hypnotic)	Gastric irritation, abdominal distention and flatulence, vertigo, ataxia, staggering gait, rashes, malaise, lightheadedness, headache, ketonuria, excitement, nightmares, delirium (especially in elderly), eosinophilia, reduction in white blood cell count and dependence on prolonged use.
Chlorambucil (Antineoplastic)	Reversible progressive lymphocytopenia and neutropenia; GI disturbances; hepatotoxicity; skin rashes; peripheral neuropathy; central neurotoxicity including seizures; interstitial pneumonia, pulmonary fibrosis. High doses may produce azoospermia and amenorrhoea and Sterility when given to boys at or before puberty.
Chloramphenicol (Antibacterial)	GI symptoms; bleeding; peripheral and optic neuritis, visual impairment, blindness; encephalopathy, confusion, delirium, mental depression, headache. Haemolysis in patients with G6PD deficiency. Ophthalmic application: Hypersensitivity reactions including rashes, fever and angioedema and Ear drops, Ototoxicity.
Chlorazepate (Hypnotics & Sedatives)	Jaundice, hepatic necrosis; extrapyramidal disorders; acute attacks of porphyria in porphyric patients, hypotension; drowsiness, fatigue, ataxia, lightheadedness, memory impairment, insomnia, anxiety, headache, depression, slurred speech, confusion, nervousness, dizziness, irritability; rash; decreased libido; xerostomia, constipation, diarrhoea, decreased salivation, nausea, vomiting, increased or decreased appetite; dysarthria, tremor; blurred vision and diplopia.

TABLE 3.2 Contd...

Name of Drugs	Adverse Drug Reactions (ADR)
Chlordiazepoxide (Anxiolytic)	Physical and psychological dependence; withdrawal syndrome; impairs psychomotor performance, aggression (in predisposed individuals especially in combination with alcohol); sedation; blood dyscrasias, jaundice and hepatic dysfunction.
Chlormethiazole (Hypnotics & Sedatives)	Nasal congestion and irritation; conjunctival irritation, headache. Rarely, paradoxical excitement, confusion, dependence, GI disturbances, rash, urticaria, bullous eruption, anaphylaxis and alterations in liver enzymes.
Chlormezanone (Muscle Relaxant)	Hypersensitivity, dizziness, diarrhoea, nausea, vomiting, renal impairment, rash and erythema multiforme.
Chloroquine (Antimalarial)	Retinopathy, hair loss, photosensitivity, tinnitus, myopathy (long-term therapy). Psychosis, seizures, leucopenia and rarely aplastic anaemia, hepatitis, GI upsets, dizziness, hypokalaemia, headache, pruritus, urticaria and difficulty in visual accommodation.
Chlorothiazide (Cardiovascular agent)	Hypotension, necrotising angiitis, dizziness, fever, headache, restlessness, vertigo, alopecia, erythema multiforme, exfoliative dermatitis, photosensitivity, purpura, rash and Stevens-Johnson syndrome.
Chlorpheniramine (Antiallergic)	Anxiety, reflex bradycardia, tachycardia, arrhythmias, headache, cold extremities/gangrene, hypertension, nausea, vomiting, sweating, weakness, fear, restlessness, insomnia, confusion, irritability, psychotic states, dyspnoea, anorexia, palpitations, extravasation causing tissue necrosis and sloughing and mydriasis.
Chlorpromazine (Anti psychotic)	Tardive dyskinesia (on long-term therapy). Involuntary movements of extremities may also occur. Dry mouth, constipation, urinary retention, mydriasis, agitation, insomnia, depression and convulsions; postural hypotension, ECG changes. Allergic skin reaction, amenorrhoea, gynaecomastia, weight gain. Hyperglycaemia and raised serum cholesterol.
Chlorpropamide (Antidiabetic)	GI disturbances (e.g. anorexia, nausea, vomiting, epigastric discomfort, abdominal cramps, constipation, and diarrhoea), vague neurologic symptoms (e.g. headache, weakness, and paraesthesia) and syndrome of inappropriate secretion of antidiuretic hormone.
Chlorprothixine (Antipsychotic)	Dry mouth, constipation, urinary retention, mydriasis; agitation, insomnia, depression, convulsions, nasal congestion, tachycardia, postural hypotension, blurred vision, inhibition of ejaculation; urticaria, exfoliative dermatitis; agranulocytosis; extrapyramidal dysfunction; altered endocrine and metabolic functions.

TABLE 3.2 Contd...

Name of Drugs	Adverse Drug Reactions (ADR)
Chlortetracycldine (Antibacterial)	Hypersensitivity and photosensitivity reactions; abnormal pigmentation of the eye; myopia
Chlorthalidone (Antihypertensive)	Orthostatic hypotension, GI disturbances, jaundice, pancreatitis, vertigo, lethargy, paraesthesia, photosensitivity, rash, muscle cramps, hypokalaemia, hyponatraemia, hyperglycaemia, hyperuricaemia or gout, leucopenia, agranulocytosis, aplastic anaemia and thrombocytopenia.
Ciaspride (Prokinetic)	Abdominal cramps, borborygmi and loose stools (transient); rarely require discontinuation of therapy. Headache
Ciclacillin (Antibiotic)	Urticaria, candida superinfection. Potentially Fatal: Anaphylactic reaction with CV collapses especially with parenteral use.
Cilazapril (Antihypertensive)	Dizziness, headache, fatigue, GI disturbances, taste disturbances, persistent dry cough and other upper respiratory tract.
Cimetidme (H_2 antagonistic)	Diarrhoea, other GI disturbances, dizziness, headache, tiredness, myalgia, arthralgia, rashes, altered LFTs, reversible confusional states. Rarely, hypersensitivity reactions and fever, reversible alopecia, blood disorders (e.g. agranulocytosis, leucopenia, and thrombocytopenia), acute pancreatitis,
Cinnarizine (Anti vertigo)	Extrapyramidal symptoms sometimes associated with severe depression. Drowsiness, headache, GI upsets, unsteadiness, headache; rarely skin and hypersensitivity reactions, dry mouth, blurred vision, urinary difficulty or retention, constipation and increased gastric reflux, fatigue and Hypolipidaemic effect.
Cinoxacin (Antibiotic)	Hypersensitivity reactions; nausea, vomiting, diarrhoea; abdominal pain; neurological effects; toxic psychoses or convulsions; skin reactions; tendon damage and hepatic effects.
Ciprofloxacin (Antibacterial)	Nausea, vomiting, diarrhoea, abdominal pain, dyspepsia; headache, dizziness, confusion, insomnia, restlessness; tremor, drowsiness, nightmares, hallucinations, psychotic reactions, depression and convulsions.
Cisplatin (Antineoplastic)	Severe nausea and vomiting. Serious toxic effects on the kidneys, bone marrows and ears. Hypomagnesaemia, hypocalcaemia, hyperuricaemia. Peripheral neuropathies, papilloedema, optic neuritis, seizures. Ototoxicity (children) manifested as tinnitus, loss of hearing, deafness or vestibular toxicity.

TABLE 3.2 Contd...

Name of Drugs	Adverse Drug Reactions (ADR)
Clarithromycin (Antibacterial)	GI upset, glossitis, stomatitis, altered taste; headache, dizziness, hallucinations, insomnia, other CNS effects; rash;
Clavulanic acid (Antibacterial)	Nausea, vomiting, diarrhoea, indigestion, rash and urticaria, candida superinfection.
Clemastine (Antiallergic)	Drowsiness, CNS depression, dizziness, sedation; diarrhoea, nausea, vomiting; blurred vision,
Clindamycin (Antibacterial)	Diarrhoea, nausea, vomiting, abdominal pain; erythema multiforme, contact dermatitis and exfoliative.
Clioquinol (Antibiotic)	Severe irritation or hypersensitivity. Cross-sensitivity with other halogenated hydroxyquinolines. May discolour fair hair.
Clobazam (Anticonvuisant)	Constipation, anorexia, nausea; dizziness, fine tremors and worsening of respiratory symptoms.
Clofazimine (Antileprotics)	Anaemia, peripheral neuropathy, haemolysis and methaemoglobinaemia (dose-related).
Clofibrate (Lipid lowening agent)	Anorexia; nausea; gastric discomfort; stomatitis; headache; dizziness; vertigo; fatigue; skin reactions andalopecia.
Clomipramine (Antidepressant)	Dryness of mouth; disturbances in micturition; drowsiness, increased sweating; sexual dysfunction and confusion.
Clomocycline (Antibiotic)	Fever, thrombophloebitis (inj). Acute anaphylactoid reactions, hyperpyrexia. Rash, erythema, pruritus, vesiculation.
Clonazepam (Anticonvuisant)	Drowsiness or sedation, fatigue, muscular hypotonia, behavioural disturbances including aggressiveness, agitation, hyperkinesis and irritability; coordination disturbances, dizziness and vertigo.
Clomdine (Antihypertensive)	Dry mouth, drowsiness, dizziness, headache, constipation, impotence, vivid dreams, urinary retention; dry, itching.
Chlorasepate (Hypnotics and sedative)	Jaundice, hepatic necrosis; extrapyramidal disorders; acute attacks of porphyria in porphyric patients,
Cloxacillin (Antibacterial)	Neutropenia, agranulocytosis; GI upsets; rash. Sore mouth or tongue. Black hairy tongue. Potentially Fatal.
Clozapine (Antipsychotic)	Drowsiness, dizziness, headache; nausea, vomiting, constipation; anxiety, confusion, fatigue and transient fever.
Cocaine (Stimulant)	Hypertension, headache, peripheral ischaemia,
Codeine (Antiillusive)	Dependence, withdrawal symptoms; nausea, vomiting, constipation, drowsiness, confusion, difficulty in micturition, ureteric or biliary spasms, urinary retention, dry mouth, dizziness, sweating, facial flushing, headache.
Colaspase (Antineoplastic)	Hypersensitivity, dizziness, diarrhoea, nausea, vomiting, renal impairment, rash and erythema multiforme,

TABLE 3.2 *Contd...*

Name of Drugs	Adverse Drug Reactions (ADR)
Colchicine (Antigout)	Nausea, vomiting and abdominal pain; diarrhoea, GI haemorrhage, rashes, renal and hepatic damage in excessive doses. Rarely peripheral neuritis, myopathy, alopecia and with chronic therapy blood disorders like agranulocytosis, aplastic anaemia.
Colistin (Antidiarrhoeal)	Acute tubular necrosis, neurotoxicity; nephrotoxicity. The neuromuscular blockade is potentially fatal, when associated with use of curariform muscle relaxants.
Cortisone (Corticosteroid)	Insomnia, nervousness, increased appetite, indigestion, hirsutism, diabetes mellitus, arthralgia, cataracts, glaucoma, epistaxis, alkalosis, Cushing's syndrome, delirium, oedema, euphoria, fractures, hallucinations,
Cyclandelate (Peripheral Vasodilator)	Flushes, GI upset, nausea, tingling, tachycardia, sweating, dizziness, headache.
Cyclizine (Antinausea/ antivertigo)	CNS depression e.g. drowsiness to deep sleep, lassitude, dizziness and incoordination.
Cyclobarbitone (Barbiturates)	Dizziness or vertigo; acute renal failure, interstitial nephritis, acute tubular necrosis; electrolyte imbalances.
Cydophosphamide (Neoplastic disorders)	Congestive heart failure; leucopenia; poor wound healing; anorexia. Nausea, vomiting; alopecia.
Cyclosertne (Antitubercular)	Headache, dizziness, anxiety, confusion, irritability, paraesthesia, speech difficulties, photosensitivity, vertigo.
Cyclosporin (Immuno depressant)	Hypertension; hepatoxicity; tremor; paraesthesia, hypertrichosis, facial oedema, acne; gingival hypertrophy.
Cyproneptadine (Antiallergic)	Confusion, disturbed coordination, dizziness, excitation, euphoria, hallucinations, headache, hysteria, insomnia, irritability, nervousness, restlessness, sedation, seizure, sleepiness, tremor, vertigo, hypotension, palpitation, tachycardia, abdominal pain, anorexia and increased appetite.
Cyproterone (Hormone)	Inhibits spermatogenesis, reduces volume of ejaculate, causes infertility, and produces abnormal spermatozoa, gynecomastia and enlargement of mammary glands; galactorrhoea and benign nodules. Depressive mood changes. Alterations in hair pattern, skin reactions. Fatigue and lassitude, breathlessness and wt changes.
Cytarabine (Neoplastic disorders)	Dementia, GI disturbances, hepatic and renal dysfunction, neurotoxicity, rashes, oral and anal ulceration, GI haemorrhage, oesophagitis, conjunctivitis, flu-like syndrome, anaphylactoid reactions.
Dacarbazine (Antineoplastic)	Impairs immune response to vaccines; possible infection after administration of live vaccines. Effect increased by CYP1A2 inhibitors e.g. amiodarone, ciprofloxacin, fluvoxamine, ketoconazole, lomefloxacin, ofloxacin and rofecoxib. Effect decreased by CYP1A2 inducers e.g. aminoglutethimide, carbamazepine, phenobarbital and rifampicin.

TABLE 3.2 Contd...

Name of Drugs	Adverse Drug Reactions (ADR)
Danazole (Gonadal hormone)	Oedema, wt gain, sweating, acne, hirsutism, flushing, oily skin or hair, deepening of the voice, clitoral hypertrophy, amenorrhoea, hepatic dysfunction, CNS or GI disturbances, benign intracranial hypertension, reduction in breast size, visual disturbances, elevated LFT values.
Dantrolen (Muscle Relaxant)	Fatigue, muscle weakness/pain. GI disturbances, CNS effects, tachycardia, unstable BP, dyspnoea, drowsiness, rashes, pruritus, chills and fever, visual disturbances, dysphagia, speech disturbances; haematuria, crystalluria, urinary frequency, retention and incontinence.
Dapsone (Antileprotic)	Anaemia, peripheral neuropathy, haemolysis and methaemoglobinaemia (dose-related), nephrotic syndrome, psychological changes, hepatitis. Others: Nausea, vomiting, anorexia, headache, maculopapular rash, toxic epidermal necrolysis, Stevens-Johnson syndrome. Topical: Dryness, redness, oiliness and peeling at application site.
Daunorubicin (Antineoplastic)	GI disturbances; stomatitis; alopoecia and dermatological reactions. Extravasation of daunorubicin may cause severe local tissue necrosis damaging surrounding muscles, tendons and nerves. IV infusion, back pain, flushing and chest tightness.
Debrisoquim	Postural hypotension, failure of ejaculation, fluid retention, nasal decongestion, headache, diarrhoea, drowsiness.
Demeclocycline (Antibacterial)	Photosensitivity, reversible nephrogenic diabetes insipidus, permanent discolouration of the teeth, brownish-black microscopic discolouration of thyroid tissue, nausea, vomiting, diarrhoea, increases in LFT values, hepatitis, jaundice, hepatic failure, rashes, pruritus, bullous dermatoses and exfoliative dermatitis.
Demethyl-chlortetracycline (Antibiotic)	Hypersensitivity, dizziness, diarrhoea, nausea, vomiting, renal impairment, rash, erythema multiforme.
Desipramine (Antidepressant)	Psychological and physical dependence,
Desmethyldiazepam (Anxiolytic)	Sedation, drowsiness, ataxia, muscle weakness, fatigue, confusion, depression, headache, vertigo, amnesia, paradoxical reactions (e.g. anxiety, hallucinations, insomnia, psychoses, sleep disturbances).
Dexamethasone (Corticosteroid)	Hypersensitivity reactions, lid itching and swelling, conjunctival erythema, increase in intraocular pressure.
Dexamphetamine (CNS stimulant)	Cardiovascular Palpitations and tachycardia.

TABLE 3.2 *Contd...*

Name of Drugs	Adverse Drug Reactions (ADR)
Dextromethorpan (Corticosteroid)	Dizziness, GI disturbances, Nausea, vomiting, dry mouth, nose and throat infection.
Dextromethorpan (Opioid analgesic)	Dizziness or vertigo and acute renal failure.
Dextropro-poxyphene (Analgesic & antipyretic)	Dizziness, sedation, nausea, vomiting and weakness.
Dezocine (Analgesic)	Nausea, vomiting, abdominal pain, diarrhoea; headache, dizziness and insomnia.
Diamorphine (Analgesic)	Hypersensitivity, dizziness, diarrhoea, nausea, vomiting, renal impairment, rash and erythema multiforme.
Diazepam (Anxiolytic)	Psychological and physical dependence with withdrawal syndrome, fatigue, drowsiness, sedation, ataxia and vertigo.
Diazoxide (Antihypertensive)	Hypotension; hyperglycaemia; oedema; dysgeusia; nausea; anorexia and other GI disturbances.
Diclofenac (NSAID agent)	GI disturbances; headache, dizziness, rash; GI bleeding, peptic ulceration; abnormalities of kidney function.
Dicloxacillin (Antibacterial)	Hypersensitivity reactions including uticaria; fever; joint pains; rashes and angioedema.
Dicoumarol (Anticoagulant)	Hypoglycaemia, nausea, epigastric fullness, heartburn, Hypoglycaemic effect enhanced by dicoumarol,
Dicyclomine (Sedative)	Dry mouth, blurred vision, irritable bowel syndrome
Didanosine (Antiviral)	Pancreatitis; peripheral neuropathy; diarrhoea, nausea, vomiting, abdominal pain; headache, fatigue and rash.
Diethylpropion (Monoamine oxidase inhibitor)	Dizziness or vertigo; acute renal failure, interstitial nephritis, acute tubular necrosis and electrolyte imbalances.
Diflunisal (Analgesic)	GI disturbances or bleeding; CNS effects; hypersensitivity reactions; blood disorders; nephrotoxicity; haematuria; oedema; pancreatitis; alveolitis; photosensitivity; pulmonary eosinophilia and pneumonitis.
Digitoxin (Cardiac glycoside)	Nausea, vomiting, anorexia, diarrhoea, abdominal pain, headache, facial pain, fatigue, weakness and dizziness.
Digoxin (Drug for heart failure)	Extra beats, anorexia, nausea and vomiting. Diarrhoea in elderly, confusion, dizziness, drowsiness, restlessness, nervousness, agitation and amnesia, visual disturbances, gynaecomastia, local irritation (IM/SC inj), rapid IV admin may lead to vasocostriction and transient hypertension.
Dihydrocodeine (Analgesic)	Nausea, vomiting, constipation, drowsiness, confusion and other CNS effects. CV effects, sweating, hypothermia.

TABLE 3.2 *Contd...*

Name of Drugs	Adverse Drug Reactions (ADR)
Dihydroergotamine (Antimigrairi)	Nausea, vomiting, diarrhoea, coronary artery vasospasm, precordial pain, numbness, cramps and localised oedema.
Dilevalol (Antihypertensive)	Orthostatic hypotension, dizziness, fatigue, vertigo, paraesthesia, headache, nasal stuffiness, dyspnoea, diarrhea.
Diltiazem (Antihypertensive)	Headache, ankle oedema, hypotension, dizziness, fatigue, flushing, nausea, GI discomfort, gingival hyperplasia.
Diphenhydramine (Antiallergic)	CNS depression, dizziness, headache, sedation; paradoxical stimulation in children and dryness of mouth.
Diphenoxylate (Antidiarrhoeal)	GI effects; headache, drowsiness, dizziness, restlessness, euphoria, depression, numbness of the extremities.
Diphenylhydantoin (Anti Convulsion Drug)	GI effects; headache, drowsiness, dizziness, restlessness, euphoria, depression, numbness of the extremities.
Diphenylpyraline (Antihistamine)	GI disturbances or bleeding; CNS effects; hyper sensitivity reactions; blood disorders; nephrotoxicity and haematuria.
Dipyridamole (Antianginal)	GI disturbances, headache, dizziness, faintness, facial flushing, skin rash, liver dysfunction, angina
Disodium Cromoglycate (Anti Asthmatic Drug)	Nausea, headache, dizziness, unpleasant taste, joint pain and swelling, skin rashes and aggravation of asthma.
Disopyramide (Antiarrhythmic)	Impotence, constipation, difficulty in micturition, dry mouth, blurred vision, nausea, bloating and abdominal pain.
Distigmine (parasympathomimetic)	Accidental trauma, fatigue, asthenia, dizziness, headache, somnolence, agitation, insomnia, confusion, depression, nausea, vomiting, diarrhoea, abdominal pain, loss of appetite, dyspepsia, upper respiratory tract infection, urinary tract infection. Rarely, angina pectoris, gastric and duodenal ulcers, GI haemorrhage; bradycardia, seizures, rashes and syncope.
Disulfiram (Antabuse)	Drowsiness, fatigue, lassitude, psychotic reactions, peripheral and optic neuropathies, hepatotoxicity, garlic-like or metallic after-taste, GI upset, body odour, bad breath, headache, impotence.
Dobutamine (Inotropic agent)	Increased Heart Rate, Blood Pressure, and Ventricular Ectopic Activity A 10- to 20-mm increase in systolic blood.
Domperidone (Antileutic)	Drowsiness, extrapyramidal reactions, galactorrhoea, gynaecomastia; constipation or diarrhea and lassitude.
Dopamine (Inotropic agent)	Nausea, vomiting, tachycardia, ectopic beats, palpitation, anginal pain, hypotension, vasoconstriction, bradycardia, hypertension, dyspnoea, headache, widened QRS complexes and azotaemia.

TABLE 3.2 *Contd...*

Name of Drugs	Adverse Drug Reactions (ADR)
Dopexamine (Synthetic dopamine analogue)	Dizziness or vertigo; acute renal failure, interstitial nephritis, acute tubular necrosis; electrolyte imbalances.
Dothiepin (Anti depressant)	Cholestatic jaundice, sexual dysfunction, exacerbation of psychotic manifestation, cardiac arrhythmias, hypotension, dry mouth.
Doxapram (Respiratory Stimulant)	Dyspnoea and other respiratory problems. Muscle involvement may range from fasciculations to spasticity.
Doxazosin (Antihypertensive)	Chest pain, fatigue, headache, influenza-like symptoms, pain, hypotension, palpitation, abdominal pain, diarrhea.
Doxepin Diflunisal	Drowsiness, dizziness, confusion, headache, dry mouth, constipation, blurring of vision, hypotension, tachycardia.
Doxycycline (Antibiotic)	Anaphylactoid reactions, Stevens-Johnson syndrome, toxic epidermal necrolysis, Clostridium difficile-associated disease (CDAD), hepatotoxicity.
Diflunisal (NSAIDs)	GI disturbances or bleeding; CNS effects; hypersensitivity reactions; blood disorders; nephrotoxicity; haematuria; oedema; pancreatitis; alveolitis; photosensitivity; pulmonary eosinophilia; pneumonitis.
Doxycycline (Antibacterial)	Permanent staining of teeth; rash, superinfection; nausea, GI upsets, glossitis; dysphagia; photosensitivity.
Droperidol (Antiemetic)	Dry mouth, constipation, micturition difficulty, blurred vision, mydriasis, delirium, agitation, catatonic-like states.
Dydrogesterone (Gonadal Hormone)	Dizziness, nausea, headache, fatigue, emotional lability, irritability; abdominal pain and distention.
Edrophonium (Miso Drug)	Muscle weakness, paralysis and muscle atrophy.
Ethosuximide (Antiseizure)	Blood toxicities and disorders; headache, fatigue, lethargy, drowsiness, dizziness, ataxia, hiccup and mild euphoria.
Emetine (Anti amoebic Drug)	Drowsiness, extrapyramidal reactions, galactorrhoea, gynaecomastia; constipation or diarrhoea, lassitude, decreased libido and skin rash.
Enalapril (Antihypertensive)	Initial hypotension may be severe and prolonged. Dizziness, headache, fatigue, persistent dry cough.
Encainide (Antiarrythmic)	Tremor, dizziness, paraesthesia, lightheadedness, nausea, vomiting, anorexia, constipation, diarrhoea, rash, blurred vision, tinnitus, lupus erythematosus, sweating, taste disturbances, liver disorders.
Enoxacin (Antibiotic)	GI disturbances; CNS effects; hypersensitivity-type reactions; reversible arthralgia; hepatic effects.
Enoxaparin (Anticoagulant)	Thrombocytopenia, mild bleeding, injection site irritation, pain and ecchymoses, hypersensitivity and erythema.

TABLE 3.2 *Contd...*

Name of Drugs	Adverse Drug Reactions (ADR)
Enoximone (Anti Heart Failure)	Fatigue, palpitations, tachycardia, nausea, diarrhea.
Epanolol (β-adrenoreceptor antagonist)	Diarrhoea, dizziness, pruritus, skin rashes, GI tract infections, chest pain, headache, nausea, pain and anxiety.
Ephednne (Respiratory agent)	Anxiety, tachycardia, tremor, dry mouth, hypertension, cardiac arrhythmias, impaired circulation to the extremities.
Epirubicin (Antineoplastic)	Myelosuppression; cardiotoxicity, alopoecia; mucositis; hyperpyrexia; lethargy; amenorrhoea; nausea and vomiting.
Ergometrine (Obstetrics Drug)	Nausea, vomiting, abdominal pain, headache, dizziness, rashes, hypertension, bradycardia and arrhythmia.
Ergonovine (Uterine Stimulant)	Nausea, vomiting, abdominal pain, diarrhoea; headache, dizziness; tinnitus; chest pain, palpitation, bradycardia, transient hypertension and other cardiac arrhythmias; dyspnoea, sometimes rashes and shock.
Ergotamine (Antimigrain)	Muscle cramps, stiffness, tiredness. Numbness and tingling of extremities. Nausea, vomiting anddiarrhea.
Erythromycin (Antibiotic)	Abdominal pain and cramping, nausea, vomiting, diarrhoea, stomatitis, heartburn, anorexia, melaena, pruritus ani, reversible mild acute pancreatitis, hepatic dysfunction, prolongation of QT interval, ventricular arrhythmias, urticaria, skin eruptions, rash, bilateral hearing loss, tinnitus, vertigo, venous irritation and thrombophlebitis.
Eserine (AntiCholinesterase inhibitor)	Dry mouth, dysphagia, constipation, flushing and dryness of skin, tachycardia, palpitations, arrhythmias and mydriasis.
Esmolol (Antiarrhythmic)	Hypotension, bradycardia, heart failure, local irritation, diaphoresis, peripheral ischaemia, dizziness and somnolence.
Estramustine (Antineoplastic)	Gynaecomastia, fluid retention and CV effects, GI disturbances, hepatic dysfunction, loss of libido, hypersensitivity.
Ethacrynic acid (Cardiovascular agent)	Fluid and electrolyte imbalance, nausea, diarrhoea, blurred vision, headache, dizziness and hypotension.
Ethambutol (Antitubercuiar drug)	Retrobulbar neuritis with a reduction in visual activity, constriction of visual field, central or peripheral scotoma.
Ethanol (Alcohol)	Loss of judgement, emotional lability, visual impairment, slurred speech and ataxia.
Ethinyloestradiol (Gonadal Hormone)	Menstrual irregularities; headache and dizziness.
Ethosuximide (Anticonvulsant)	Blood toxicities and disorders; headache, fatigue, lethargy, drowsiness, dizziness, ataxia, hiccup and mild euphoria.

TABLE 3.2 *Contd...*

Name of Drugs	Adverse Drug Reactions (ADR)
Etidocaine (Anaesthetic)	Dizziness, paraesthesia, drowsiness and confusion.
Etintidine (Antispasmodic)	Nausea, vomiting, dry mouth, constipation and allergic reactions.
Ethyl biscoumacetate (Anticoagulant)	Headache, asthenia, tremor, palpitations, nausea and diarrhea.
Etodolac (NSAID)	Acute renal failure; blood disorder; nephrotoxicity; angioedema, arrhythmia, bone marrow suppression, CHF, dyspnoea, erythema multiforme, exfoliative dermatitis, hepatitis, hypertension, peripheral neuropathy, Stevens-Johnson syndrome, syncope, tachycardia, toxic amblyopia, toxic epidermal necrolysis and urticaria.
Etomodate (Anaesthetic agent)	Excitatory phenomena Example, involuntary myoclonic muscle movements, convulsions; hypersensitivity reactions, pain on injection; post operative nausea and vomiting.
Etoposide (Antineoplastic agent)	Nausea, vomiting, anorexia, diarrhoea, stomatitis; reversible alopoecia; rarely, disturbances of liver dysfunction.
Famciclovir (Antiviral)	Dizziness, headache, diarrhoea, constipation, nausea, vomiting, hallucinations, confusion and pruritus.
Famotidine (H_2 antagonist)	Headache, dizziness, constipation, diarrhoea, nausea, rash, GI discomfort, fatigue, gynaecomastia and impotence.
Felbamate (Antiseizure agent)	Somnolence, headache, fever, dizziness, insomnia, fatigue, nervousness, anorexia, nausea, vomiting and constipation.
Felodipine (Anti hypertensive)	Flushing, headache, peripheral oedema, tachycardia, palpitation, dizziness, fatigue. Ankle swelling.
Fenbufen (Antiinflammatory)	GI disorder; skin rashes; CNS disorders; erythema multiforme; photosensitivity; haematuria; renal failure (rarely); pulmonary eosinophilia or an allergic and aplastic alveolitis. Haemolytic anaemia.
Fenfluramine (Monoamine)	Convulsions; liver damage; shivering; nausea; vomiting; involuntary muscle movements; hiccup; coughing; bronchospasm; laryngospasm; hypotension; cardiac arrhythmias; respiratory depression; mild hypothermia; malignant hyperthermia; uterine relaxation (high concentrations); hypotension; asthma.
Fenoprofen (Antiinflammatory)	GI disorders, cholestatic jaundice, occult blood in stools; headache; itching; fluid retention; dizziness and somnolence.
Fenoterol (Respiratory agent)	Fine tremor of skeletal muscle, palpitations, tachycardia, nervous tension, headachesand peripheral vasodilatation.

TABLE 3.2 *Contd...*

Name of Drugs	Adverse Drug Reactions (ADR)
Fentanyl (Neuromuscular blocker)	Nausea, vomiting; bradycardia, oedema, CNS depression, confusion, dizziness, drowsiness, headache and sedation.
Finasteride (Urogenital/ Antispasmodic)	Testicular pain. Hypersensitivity reactions e.g. swelling of lips and face, urticaria and rashes.
Flecamide (Antiarrythemic)	Dizziness, visual disturbances, lightheadedness and other CNS effects, nausea, vomiting, headache and tremor.
Floxuridine (Antineoplastic)	Ophthalmic: Irritation; inflammation of the eye or eyelids; pain; photophobia; pruritus; conjunctivitis; oedema. Rarely, lachrymal duct occlusion and hypersensitivity reactions. Corneal damage (prolonged use). Topical: Irritation; stinging; hypersensitivity reactions; corneal punctate defects or skin maceration (when applied excessively).
Flucloxacillin (Antibiotic)	Hypersensitivity reactions including urticaria; fever; joint pains; rashes; angioedema; serum sickness-like reactions.
Fluconazole (Antifungal)	Nausea, abdominal pain, vomiting, diarrhoea, flatulence; elevated liver function values; headache and rash.
Flucytosine (Antiinflammatory)	GI symptoms e.g. nausea, vomiting, diarrhoea. Skin rashes, hypokalaemia, peripheral neuropathy and headache.
Fludrocortisone (Corticosteroid)	Hypertension, sodium and water retention, potassium loss, dizziness, itching, skin rash, headache and convulsions.
Flufenamic acid (Anti inflammatory)	Abdominal pain, dyspepsia, constipation, diarrhoea, nausea, GI ulcers; oedema; bronchospasm and headache.
Flumazenil (Misc. Drug)	Nausea, vomiting, dizziness, blurred vision, headache, flushing; anxiety, fear and agitation.
Flunitrazepam (Anxiolytic)	Drowsiness and lightheadedness, sedation, muscle weakness and ataxia and less frequently vertigo.
5-Fluorouracil (Antineoplastic)	Leucopenia, thrombocytopaenia, stomatitis, GI ulceration, bleeding and diarrhoea, haemorrhage from any site (stop treatment). Nausea, vomiting, rashes, hyperpigmentation, alopecia. Topical: Local inflammatory and photosensitivity reactions. Dermatitis and erythema multiforme (rare).
Fluoxetine (Antidepressant)	Nervousness, insomnia, anxiety, headache, tremor, drowsiness, dry mouth, nausea, vomiting, sweating and diarrhea.
Flupenthixol (Antipsychotic)	Rigidity, tremors, restlessness, tardive dyskinesia, insomnia, dryness of mouth, wt gain and sexual dysfunction.
Fluphenazine (Antipsychotic)	Tardive dyskinesia, sedation, mental confusion; hypotension; hyperprolactinaemia leading to galactorrhoea.
Flurazepam (Hypnotic)	Drowsiness and lightheadedness, sedation, muscle weakness and ataxia; less frequently vertigo and headache.

TABLE 3.2 *Contd...*

Name of Drugs	Adverse Drug Reactions (ADR)
Flurbiprofen (NSAID agent)	Fluid retention, oedema; allergic nephritis, allergic reactions; GI upsets; dizziness, tinnitus.
Fluspirilene (Antipsychotic)	Parkinsonian symptoms, dystonia, akathisia, tardive dyskinesia. Interference with temp regulation. Neuroleptic.
Flutamide (Antineoplastic agent)	Hot flushes, loss of libido, impotence, gynaecomastia, nausea, vomiting, diarrhea and increased appetite.
Foscarnet (Antiviral)	Diarrhoea, nausea, vomiting and abdominal pain.
Fosfomycin (Antibiotic)	GI disturbances, transient increases in serum concentrations of aminotransferases; headache and visual disturbances.
Fosinopril (ACE inhibitor)	Dizziness, orthostatic hypotension, palpitation, headache, weakness, fatigue, hyperkalaemia, chest pain.
Frusemide (Diuretics)	Fluid and electrolyte imbalance, nausea, diarrhoea, blurred vision, headache, dizziness, hypotension, photosensitisation, hepatic dysfunction, hyperglycaemia and glycosuria, rarely bone marrow depression, gynaecomastia, hirsutism, hoarseness, menstrual irregularities, loss of libido and impotence.
Fusidic acid (Antibacterial)	Jaundice and liver dysfunction (reversible); GI disturbances. IV: Venospasm, thrombophloebitis and haemolysis.
Gabapentin (Anticonvulsant)	Somnolence, dizziness, ataxia, weakness, paraesthesia, fatigue, headache; nystagmus, diplopia; nausea and vomiting.
Gallopamil (Calcium antagonist)	Rarely, nausea or vertigo, headache, hypotension, dizziness, flushing, bradycardiac arrhythmias, CHF and AV block.
Ganciclovir (Antiviral)	Haematolgical disturbances; marrow depression; GI disturbances; fever, rash and abnormal LFTs; irritation.
Gemfibrozil (Lipid lowering agent)	Myositic syndrome, cholelithiasis, GI disturbances, rash, headache, blood dyscrasias.
Gentamicm (Antibacterial/ Antifungal)	Dizziness or vertigo; acute renal failure, interstitial nephritis, acute tubular necrosis; electrolyte imbalance.
Glibenclamide (Oral Antidiabetic)	Serum levels may be reduced by colesevelam. May increase hypoglycaemic effect w/ MAOIs, chloramphenicol, fluoroquinolones (e.g. ciprofloxacin), probenecid, NSAIDs, ACE inhibitors and fluoxetine.
Glibornuride (Anti diabetic)	GI disturbances; metallic taste; skin rashes, pruritus, and photosensitivity; facial flushing and hypoglycaemia.
Gliclazide (Oral Antidiabetic)	GI disturbances, skin reaction, leucopenia, thrombocytopenia, agranulocytosis, haemolytic anaemia and cholestati.

TABLE 3.2 *Contd...*

Name of Drugs	Adverse Drug Reactions (ADR)
Glipizide (Oral Antidiabetic)	GI upsets, diarrhoea, nausea; allergic skin reactions, leucopenia, thrombocytopenia, agranulocytosis.
Gliquidone (Anti diabetic)	GI disturbances; metallic taste; skin rashes, pruritus, and photosensitivity; facial flushing and hypoglycaemia.
Glutethimide (Hypotonic sedative)	Orthostatic hypotension, dizziness, fatigue, vertigo, paraesthesia and headache.
Glyburide (Antidiabetic)	Blood dyscrasias (reversible), liver dysfunction, hypoglycaemia, GI symptoms, allergic skin reactions
Glyceryltn (Antianginal/ coronary vasodilator)	Facial flushing, dizziness, tachycardia, throbbing headache and tolerance. Large doses can cause vomiting, Headache, nausea, diarrhoea, thirst, mental confusion.
Glycopyrronium (Antisparmodic)	Xerostomia; loss of taste, nausea, vomiting, constipation, reduced sweating; urinary hesitancy and retention.
Glymidine (Antidiabetic)	Fluid and electrolyte disorders e.g. acidosis, electrolyte loss, marked diuresis, urinary retention, and oedema.
Goserelin (Hormone)	Vaginal bleeding and dryness, arthralgia, paraesthesias, increase in menstrual bleeding and hot flushes.
Gold sodium (Thiomalate)	Skin and mucous membrane reactions; stomatitis with a metallic taste; rash with pruritus.
Granisetron (Antiemetic)	Headache; sensation of flushing; constipation; hypersensitivity reactions; chest pain; dizziness.
Griseofulvin (Antifungal)	Oral thrush; GI distress, taste perversion; dizziness, confusion, headache, depression, insomnia and fatigue.
Guanabenz (Antihypertensive)	Weight Gain, Dizziness, orthostatic hypotension, palpitation, headache, weakness, Fatigue, hyperkalaemia and chest pain.
Guanadrel (Antihypertensive)	Cardiac abnormalities and hypertension.
Guanethidine (Antihypertensive)	Severe postural and exertional hypotension, diarrhoea, dizziness, syncope, muscle weakness, lassitude and angina.
Guanfecine (Antihypertensive)	Drowsiness, dry mouth, dizziness, headache, constipation, depression, anxiety, fatigue, nausea, anorexia, parotid pain, sleep disturbances, vivid dreams, impotence and loss of libido, urinary retention or incontinence, slight orthostatic hypotension and fluid retention.
Guanoxan (Anti-hypertensive)	Dizziness or vertigo; acute renal failure, interstitial nephritis, acute tubular necrosis and electrolyte imbalances.
Haloperidol (Antipsychotic)	Tardive dyskinesia; extrapyramidal reactions. Anxiety, drowsiness, depression, anorexia, transient tachycardia.

TABLE 3.2 *Contd...*

Name of Drugs	Adverse Drug Reactions (ADR)
Heparin (Anticoagulant, Antithrombosis)	Slight fever, headache, chills, nausea, vomiting, constipation, epistaxis, bruising, slight haematuria, skin necrosis.
Heroin (Opoid Analgesic)	Nausea, vomiting, dry mouth, constipation and allergic reactions.
Hexobarbital (Hypnotic)	GI disturbances, visual impairment and irritation;serum concentrations of digoxin, ciclosporin and terfenadine.
Homatropine (Anticholinergic Drug)	Blurred vision; photophobia; increased intraocular pressure. Prolonged use may cause local irritation characterized by follicular conjunctivitis, vascular congestion, oedema, and exudate and eczematoid dermatitis.
Hydralazine (Antihypertensive)	Tachycardia; palpitations; angina pectoris; haemolytic anaemia; paralytic ileus; severe headache and GI disturbances.
Hydrochlorothiazide (Diuretic)	Volume depletion and electrolyte imbalance, dry mouth, thirst, lethargy, drowsiness, muscle pain and cramps.
Hexobarbital (Sedative)	GI disturbances, visual impairment and irritation; serum concentrations of digoxin, ciclosporin and terfenadine.
Hydralazine (Antihypertensive)	Tachycardia; palpitations; angina pectoris; haemolytic anaemia; paralytic ileus; severe headache and GI disturbances.
Hydrochlorothiazide (Diuretic)	Volume depletion and electrolyte imbalance, dry mouth, thirst, lethargy, drowsiness and muscle pain.
Hydralazine (Antihypertensive)	Tachycardia; palpitations; angina pectoris; haemolytic anaemia; paralytic ileus; severe headache and GI disturbances.
Hydrochlorothiazide (Diuretic)	Volume depletion and electrolyte imbalance, dry mouth, thirst, lethargy, drowsiness, muscle pain and cramps.
Hydrochlorothiazide (Diuretic)	Nebivolol Headache, fatigue, parasthesias, dizziness, dry mouth, thirst, lethargy, drowsiness, muscle pain and cramps.
Hydrocortisone (Corticosteroid)	Sodium and fluid retention. Potassium and calcium depletion. Muscle wasting, weakness, osteoporosis.
Hydroxizine (Anxiolytic, Sedatives)	CNS depression, paradoxical CNS stimulation, dry mouth, thickened respiratory secretions and constipation.
Hydroxychloroquine (Antiprotozoal)	Retinopathy, hair loss, photosensitivity, tinnitus, Psychosis and seizures.
Hydroxyprogesterone (Gonadal Hormone)	GI disturbances, increased appetite, wt gain or loss, oedema, acne, allergic skin rashes and urticaria.
Hydroxyurea (Antineoplastic)	GI disturbances, renal impairment, pulmonary oedema, dermatological reactions, headache and dizziness.

TABLE 3.2 *Contd...*

Name of Drugs	Adverse Drug Reactions (ADR)
Hydroxzine (Anti Histamine)	CNS depression, paradoxical CNS stimulation, dry mouth, thickened respiratory secretions and constipation.
Hyoscine (Antinausea)	Flushing, postural hypotension, tachycardia, fibrillation. Rarely psychotic reactions and Dizziness.
Ibuprofen (NSAID agent)	Dyspepsia, vomiting, abdominal pain, heart burn, nausea, diarrhoea, epigastric pain, edema and fluid retention.
Idoxuridine (Antinausea)	Irritation; inflammation of the eye or eyelids; pain; photophobia; pruritus; conjunctivitis and oedema.
Ifosfamide (Antineoplastic)	Confusion, alopoecia, nausea, vomiting, phloebitis, somnolence, depression and hallucinations.
Imipenem (Antibiotic)	Skin rashes, urticaria, eosinophilia, fever, nausea, vomiting, diarrhoea, and tooth or tongue discoloration.
Imipramine (Antidepressant)	Sinus tachycardia, AV/bundle-branch block, postural hypotension, dry mouth, wt loss/gain and constipation.
Indapamide (Antihypertensive)	Headache, dizziness, weakness, drowsiness, fatigue, agitation, nervousness, anorexia, nausea, vomiting and pain.
Indomethacin (NSAID agent)	Dyspepsia, nausea, abdominal pain, and diarrhea. Constipation, anorexia, flatulence and gastroenteritis.
Indoramine (α-adreno receptor antagonist)	Rash, pruritus, urticaria, dyspepsia, nausea, peptic ulcer disease, headache, dizziness and insomnia.
Interferon (Antiviral)	Depressive illness, suicidal behaviour, irritability, insomnia, anxiety. Flu-like symptoms and Headache.
Interferon (Antiviral)	Flu-like symptoms; alopecia; hypersensitivity reactions; nausea; anorexia and myelosuppression;
Indoramin (α-1 adreno receptor antagonist)	Loss of judgement, emotional lability and visual impairment.
Insulin (Pancreatic Hormone)	Hypoglycaemia, insulin resistance, lipoatrophy, oedema; pruritus and rash.
Ipratropium (Antiasthamatic)	Dry mouth, urinary retention, buccal ulceration, paralytic ileus, headache, nausea and constipation.
Iprindole (AntiDepressant)	Hypersensitivity, dizziness, diarrhoea, nausea, vomiting, renal impairment, rash, erythema multiforme.
Iproniazid (Monoamine oxidase inhibitor)	Skin rash, urticaria; eosinophilia, diarrhoea, nausea, vomiting; phloebitis; hypoprothrombinaemia and superinfection.
Isocarboxazid (Monoamine oxidase inhibitor)	Vertigo; acute renal failure, interstitial nephritis, acute tubular necrosis; electrolyte imbalances, dizziness, diarrhoea, nausea, vomiting, renal impairment and rash.

TABLE 3.2 *Contd...*

Name of Drugs	Adverse Drug Reactions (ADR)
Isoniazid (Antituberculars)	Peripheral neuritis, optic neuritis; psychotic reactions, convulsions, nausea, vomiting, fatigue and epigastric distress.
Isoprenaline (Antiasthamatic)	Nervousness, restlessness, insomnia, anxiety, tension, blurring of vision, fear, excitement.
Isosorbide dinitrate (Antianginal)	Hypotension, tachycardia, flushing, headache, dizziness, palpitation, syncope, confusion. Nausea and vomiting.
Isosorbide mononitrate (Antianginal)	Hypotension, tachycardia, flushing, headache, dizziness, palpitation, syncope, confusion and Nausea.
Isoxsuprine (Peripheral Vasodilator)	Hypotension, dizziness, palpitation, nausea, vomiting, abdominal distress, severe rash, flushing and tachycardia.
Isotretinoin (Anti-acne)	Dryness of mucous membranes, dryness of skin with scaling, fragility, erythema, cheilitis and pruritus.
Isradipine (Calcium antagonist)	Dizziness; flushing; headache; hypotension; peripheral oedema; tachycardia; palpitations and GI disturbances.
Itraconazole (Antifungal)	Dyspepsia, abdominal pain, nausea, vomiting, diarrhoea; menstrual disorders; constipation, rash and pruritus.
Kanamycin (Antibacterial)	Pain, inflammation, bruising, haematoma at injection site; GI disturbances; malabsorption of fat and loose feces.
Ketamine (Anaesthetics)	severe confusion, hallucinations, unusual thoughts, extreme fear, Less serious side effects may include,
Ketanserin (Antihypertensive)	Sedation, fatigue, lightheadedness, dizziness, headache, dry mouth, GI disturbances and oedema.
Ketazolam (Sedative)	Diarrhoea, depression, sedation, hyperacusis, rebound, insomnia, tension, photophobia and severe anxiety.
Ketoconazole (Antifungal)	GI disturbances e.g. nausea and vomiting; rash, dermatitis, burning sensation, pruritus; headache, dizziness and allergic reactions.
Ketoprofen (NSAIDs)	HTN; GI symptoms e.g. dyspepsia, discomfort, nausea, diarrhoea; pain and tissue damage at injection site (IM).
Ketorolac (Analgesic & antipyretic)	Swelling of face, fingers, lower legs, ankles, feet, weight gain, Bruising, high blood pressure, skin rash or itching.
Labetalol (Antihypertensive)	Orthostatic hypotension, dizziness, fatigue, vertigo, paraesthesia, headache, nasal stuffiness, dyspnoea and diarrhea.
Lanatoside C (Cardiovascular agent)	Nausea, vomiting, anorexia, diarrhoea, abdominal pain, headache, facial pain, fatigue, weakness and dizziness.
Latamoxef (Antibiotic)	Hypoprothrombinaemia, serious bleeding episodes, fever, pain at inj site, diarrhea and cutaneous eruption.

TABLE 3.2 Contd...

Name of Drugs	Adverse Drug Reactions (ADR)
Leucovorin (Antineoplastics)	Allergic sensitization, including anaphylactoid reactions, urticaria, GI toxicity, seizures, syncope and hypersensitivity.
Levallorphan (Opoid Antidote)	Respiratory depression, apnea, rigidity, and bradycardia, respiratory arrest, circulatory depression,
Levamisole (Anthelmintic)	Nausea, vomiting, diarrhoea, abdominal pain, dizziness and headache, fever, influenza-like syndrome and arthralgia.
Levobunolol (Antiglucoma)	Ocular stinging, burning, blepharoconjunctivitis, decreased heart rate, decreased BP, iridocyclitis and headache.
Levodopa (Antirigidity/antitremor)	Abnormal thinking, agitation, anxiety, clenching or grinding of teeth, clumsiness or unsteadiness.
Levorphanol (Analgesic)	Nausea, vomiting, constipation, dizziness, headache, fatigue, dry mouth, sweating, itching and allergic reaction.
Levonorgestrel (Birth Control)	Menstrual irregularities; headache, dizziness; breast discomfort; gynaecomastia; depression.
Lidoflazine (Antianginal)	First-degree AV block, drowsiness, dizziness and headaches.
Lignocain (Anaesthetics)	Flushing, redness of the skin, small red or purple spots on the skin, swelling at the site of application.
Lincornycin (Antibacterial)	Hypotension (IV); vertigo; dermatitis, erythema multiforme, rash, urticaria; colitis, diarrhoea, glossitis and nausea.
Liothyroine (Thiroid agent)	Arm, back or jaw pain, changes in appetite, chest pain, chest tightness, cold clammy skin, confusion and diarrhea.
Lisinopril (Antihypertensive)	Kidney disease, liver disease, heart disease or congestive heart failure, diabetes, Marfan syndrome.
Lisuride (antiparkinson drug)	Confusion, drowsiness, delirium, memory disturbance and visual hallucination.
Lithium (Antidepressant)	Heart disease, kidney disease, underactive thyroid, hyponatremia.
Lofepramine (Antidepressants)	Hypotension, cardiac arrhythmias, convulsion, coma, urinary retension, palpitations and metabolic acidosis.
Lomefloxacin (Antibacterial)	Nausea, abdominal pain or discomfort, diarrhoea; headache, dizziness, insomnia; rash, pruritus and photosensitivity.
Loperamide (Antidiarrhoeal)	Bloating, constipation, loss of appetite, stomach pain, nausea and vomiting and skin rash.
Loracarbef (Cephalosporin antibiotics)	Diarrhoea, nausea, vomiting, abdominal pain; headache; skin rashes; abnormalities in haematological parameters.
Loratidine (Antiallergic)	Diarrhea, epistaxis, pharyngitis, flu-like symptoms, fatigue, stomatitis, tooth disorder, Headache, somnolence, fatigue and dry mouth.

TABLE 3.2 Contd...

Name of Drugs	Adverse Drug Reactions (ADR)
Lorazepam (Sedative)	Drowsiness, relaxed, calm, sleepiness, abdominal pain, aggressive, angry, agitation, anxiety, attack, assault, or force, black, tarry stools.
Lorcainide (Antiarrythmic)	Mild insomnia, sudden cardiac death and convulsions.
Lormustine (Antineoplastic)	Pulmonary infiltrates, pulmonary fibrosis, nausea, vomiting, hepatotoxicity, nephrotoxicity, stomatitis and alopecia.
Lornoxicam (Antiinflammatory)	Abdominal pain, diarrhoea, dizziness, dyspepsia, nausea, vomiting; headache and haematologic disorders.
Lovastatin (Lipid lowering agent)	Bladder pain, cloudy urine, chest tightness, cough, painful urination, difficulty with moving, fever, headache and joint pain.
Lymecycline (Antiinflammatory)	GI disturbances, hypersensitivity and photosensitivity.
Lysergide (Recreational Drug)	Rhabdomyolysis, renal failure and prolonged mania.
Maprotiline (Antidepressants)	Vomiting, epigastric distress, diarrhea, bitter taste, tingling, motor hyperactivity, akathisia, seizures, restlessness, nightmares, hypomania.
Mazindol (Monoarnine oxidase inhibitor)	Nervousness, agitation, dizziness, drowsiness, depression, psychosis, vertigo, insomnia and dryness of mouth.
Mebendazole (Anthelmintics)	Nausea, vomiting, diarrhea, and abdominal pain, Rash, pruritus and urticaria.
Mecamyramine (Anti Hypertention)	Nausea, vomiting, anorexia, glossitis, and dryness of mouth, dizziness, postural hypotension, convulsions, choreiform movement and tremor.
Mecillinam (Antibiotic)	Hypersensitivity reactions including angioedema, urticaria, rash, serum sickness-like reactions and haemolytic anemia.
Meclizine (Antihistamine, H₁ antagonist)	Drowsiness, dry mouth and blurred vision.
Medazepam (Anxiolytic)	Fatigue, drowsiness, dizziness, prolonged reaction time, headache, coordination disorders, confusion.
Medifoxamine (Antidepressant)	Hypertension, hypotension, hyperprolactinaemia leading to galactorrhea, constipation, depression, headache.
Medigoxin (Cardiac glycoxide)	Extra beats, anorexia, nausea and vomiting. Diarrhoea in elderly, confusion, dizziness, drowsiness and restlessness.
Medroxy-progesterone (Gonadai Hormone)	Depression, fluid retention, fatigue, insomnia, dizziness, headache, nausea, breast tenderness and wt gain/loss.

TABLE 3.2 *Contd...*

Name of Drugs	Adverse Drug Reactions (ADR)
Mefenamic acid (Analgesic, antipyretic)	Abdominal pain, dyspepsia, constipation, diarrhoea, nausea, GI ulcers, oedema, bronchospasm and headache.
Mefloquin (Antimalanal)	Dizziness, myalgia, nausea, fever, headache, vomiting, chills, diarrhea, skin rash, abdominal pain and fatigue.
Mefruside (Diuretic)	Electrolyte imbalance, hyperglycaemia; gout, dry mouth, thirst, weakness, muscle pain and cramp and seizures.
Mepacrine (Anti Protozoal Drug)	Dizziness, headache; nausea, vomiting, reversible yellow discolouration of the skin and conjunctiva.
Meperidine (Analgesic)	Weakness, headache, disorientation, respiratory depression, delirium, seizures, tremors and dizziness,
Melphalan (Antineoplastic)	Diarrhoea, stomatitis, vomiting; haemolytic anaemia, vasculitis, pulmonary fibrosis, hepatic disorders.
Mepacaine (Antimalarial)	Dizziness, headache; nausea, vomiting; reversible yellow discolouration of the skin, conjunctiva, psychosis, CNS stimulation, convulsions.
Mepenzolate (Antispasmodic)	Dizziness, drowsiness, headache, weakness, nausea, vomiting, constipation, bloatedness, weakness and loss of taste.
Mepivacaine (Anaesthetic)	Hives, itching, skin redness, nausea, sweating, feeling hot, fast heartbeats, sneezing, difficult breathing.
Meprobamate (Hypnotic)	Drowsiness, blurred vision, diarrhea, dizziness, false sense of well-being, headache, nausea, vomiting, unusual tiredness and weakness.
Meptazinol (Analgesic)	Nausea, vomiting, constipation, diarrhoea, stomach pains, indigestion, dizziness, vertigo and drowsiness.
Mercaptopurine (Antineoplastic)	Nausea, vomiting, anorexia, diarrhea, skin rashes, alopecia, and hyperpigmentation.
Mesalazine (Antiinflammatory)	Abdominal pain, eructation, nausea, diarrhea, dyspepsia, ulcerative colitis, vomiting, constipation.
Metaraminol (Cardiovascular agent)	Apprehension, anxiety, restlessness, tremor, weakness, faintness, dizziness, headache and precordial pain.
Metformin (Oral antidiabetic)	Vomiting, abdominal pain, nausea, dyspnea, hypothermia, hypotension, and bradycardia, flatulence and abdominal pain.
Methadone (Respiratory agent)	Confusion, disorientation, dysphoria, euphoria, seizures, sleepiness or insomnia, and dizziness and confusion.
Methaqualone (Hypnotic)	Dizziness, nausea, vomiting, diarrhea, abdominal cramps, fatigue, itching, rashes, sweating, dry mouth, headache, insomnia and tremors.

TABLE 3.2 *Contd...*

Name of Drugs	Adverse Drug Reactions (ADR)
Methicillin (Antibiotic)	Neutropenia, leukopenia, thrombocytopenia, rash, eosinophilia, pruritus, fever, chills, and myalgias and pain at injection site.
Methimazole (Anti Thyroid)	Stomach upset, nausea, vomiting, mild rash, headache, drowsiness, dizziness, nausea, vomiting, or stomach upset, itching and minor skin rash.
Methocarbamol (Muscle Relaxant)	Diarrhea, difficulty swallowing, dizziness, fast heartbeat, feeling of warmth, fever, headache, itching and joint or muscle pain.
Methohexitone (Anaesthetic)	Gangrene, Thrombosis, Bronchospasm, Cardiovascular collapse and Local pain.
Methotrexate (Antineoplastic)	Nausea, vomiting, diarrhea, pharyngitis, stomatitis, anorexia, hematemesis, melena, gastrointestinal ulceration and bleeding, enteritis.
Methoxamine (Anti Hypotensive Drug)	Excessive BP elevations particularly with high dosage, ventricular ectopic beats, reflex bradycardia nausea.
Methotrimeprazine (Antipsychotic)	Drowsiness, dry mouth or constipation, dry mouth and skin rash.
Methylamphetamine (CNS Stimulation)	Dry mouth, unpleasant taste, diarrhea, constipation, anorexia, weight loss, restlessness, dizziness, insomnia, euphoria, dyskinesia, dysphoria, tremor and headache.
Methyldopa (Antihypertensive)	Slow heart rate, yellowed skin, fever, confusion or weakness, nausea, upper stomach pain and itching,
Methylphenobarbitone (Barbiturates)	Dizziness, clumsiness, sleepiness, staggering walk, drowsiness, vomiting, tiredness and nausea.
Methylprednisolone (Corticosteroid)	Hypokalemia, ulceration, insomnia to nervousness, restlessness, mania, catatonia, depression, delusions, hallucinations and violent behavior.
Methyltestosterone (Hormone)	Oedema, headache, anxiety, depression; acne, male-pattern baldness, seborrhea and hypercalcaemia.
Methyprylone (Barbiturates)	Ataxia, dysarthria, vertigo and dizziness.
Methysergide (Analgesic)	Malaise, fatigue, weight loss, backache, low grade fever, urinary obstruction, dyspnea, tightness, pain in the chest, insomnia and drowsiness.
Metoclopramide (Prokinetic)	Extrapyramidal symptoms, restlessness, drowsiness, anxiety, diarrhoea, hypotension, hypertension and headache.
Metocurine (Muscle relaxant)	Allergic reactions.
Metolazone (Diuretic)	Chest pain, palpitation, necrotising angiitis, orthostatic hypotension, syncope, venous thrombosis and vertigo.

TABLE 3.2 *Contd...*

Name of Drugs	Adverse Drug Reactions (ADR)
Metoprolol (Antihypertensive)	Asthma, COPD, sleep apnea, liver disease, congestive heart failure, problems with circulation, thyroid disorder, pheochromocytoma.
Metronidazole (Antibacterial/antifungal)	Convulsive seizures, encephalopathy, aseptic meningitis, Headache, dizziness, omitting and abdominal discomfort.
Mexiletine (Antiarrythmatic)	Dysphagia, salivary changes, altered taste, changes in oral mucosa, hiccups, peptic ulcer disease, tremor, dizziness, and difficulties with coordination.
Mezlocillin (Antibiotic)	Diarrhoea, nausea, vomiting, pseudomembranous enterocolitis and hypersensitivity reactions.
Mianserin (Antidepressant)	Drowsiness, liver dysfunction and jaundice, gynaecomastia; convulsions, hypomania, hypotension and hypertension.
Miconazole (Antibacterial/ antifungal)	Oral discomfort, oral pain, dry mouth, glossodynia, loss of taste, altered taste, tongue ulceration, mouth ulceration and tooth disorder.
Midazolam (Anxiolytic)	Nausea, vomiting, and hiccups, alterations in blood pressure, arrhythmias and ventricular irritability.
Midodrine (Antihypertensive)	Cardiac awareness, pounding in the ears, headache, and blurred vision, dizziness, skin hyperesthesia and insomnia.
Milrinone (Phosphodiesterase-3 inhibitor)	Ventricular arrhythmias, sustained and nonsustained ventricular tachycardia, ventricular & arterial fibrillation, headaches, tremor and dizziness.
Mifepristone (Antiprogesterone)	Uterine cramping, uterine hemorrhage, vaginitis, leukorrhea, pelvic pain, abdominal pain, nausea, vomiting, diarrhea, dyspepsia.
Minocycline (Antibacterials)	Liver disease, kidney disease, asthma and sulfite allergy.
Minoxidil (Antihypertensive vasodilator)	Sinus tachycardia, provocation of angina, edema, weight gain, nausea and vomiting, contact dermatitis, desquamative, bullous rashes.
Misonidazole (Radiosencitizer)	Hypotension, nausea and vomiting.
Misoprstol (prostaglandin analog)	Diarrhoea, abdominal pain, dyspepsia, constipation, flatulence, nausea, vomiting, abnormal vaginal bleeding.
Mitomycin (Antineoplastic)	Hemolytic-uremic syndrome, microangiopathic hemolytic anemia, nephropathy and marrow depression.
Mitotane (Antineoplastic)	Anorexia, nausea, vomiting, diarrhea, hypersialorrhea, dizziness, vertigo, weakness, muscle tremors and headache.
Mitozantrone (Antineoplastic)	Arrhythmia, oedema, ECG changes, pain, fatigue, fever, headache; alopecia, nail bed changes and amenorrhoea.

TABLE 3.2 Contd...

Name of Drugs	Adverse Drug Reactions (ADR)
Moclobemide (Monoamine oxidase inhibitor)	Tachycardia, hypotension, dizziness, headache, drowsiness, sleep disturbances, agitation, nervousness and sedation.
Molindone (Antipsychotic)	Orthostatic hypotension, tachycardia, arrhythmia; extrapyramidal *reactions*, mental depression.
Monosialoganglioside (A ganglioside)	Existing attitudes, nausea and vomiting.
Morocizine (Antiarrythemic)	Atrial and ventricular arrhythmias, heart failure, hypotension, syncope, vomiting or diarrhea, abdominal discomfort, anxiety, fatigue.
Morphine (Analgesic, antipyretic)	Convulsions, nausea, vomiting, dry mouth, constipation, urinary retention, headache, vertigo and palpitations.
Moxalactam (Antibiotic)	Vomiting, headache, dizziness, oral vaginal candidiasis, pseudomembranous colitis.
Mustine (Antineoplastic)	Nausea and vomiting are dose-limiting. Anorexia and diarrhea have also been reported. Hypersensitivity side effects and cardiac irregularities.
Nabilone (Antinausea)	Nasal congestion and irritation and conjunctival irritation.
Nabumetone (NSAIDs)	Drowsiness, insomnia; reduced sexual ability; bradycardia, palpitation, oedema, CHF and reduced peripheral.
Nadolol (β-adrenoreceptor antagonist)	Hypersensitivity reactions, local reactions, renal, hepatic, or nervous system effects with high dosage.
Nafcillin (Antibiotic)	Nausea and epigastric pain, rash, hepatitis or hepatic failure, hearing loss.
Naftidrofuryl (Cerebral vasodialator)	Chest pain, difficult breathing, difficulty swallowing, fainting, fast, pounding and irregular heartbeat.
Nalbuphine (Analgesic)	Sedation, dizziness, vertigo, miosis, headache; nausea, vomiting, dry mouth; itching, burning, urticaria.
Nalidixic acid (Antibacterial)	Nausea, vomiting, diarrhoea, abdominal pain; photosensitivity reactions, allergic rash, urticaria, pruritus and visual disturbances.
Nalorphine (Opoid Antidote)	Drowsiness, respiratory depression, miosis, dysphoria and lethargy.
Naloxone (Antipoisoning)	Stomach cramps, body aches, convulsions, diarrhea, difficult breathing, excessive crying, fast, pounding, irregular heartbeat and fever.
Naltrexone (Antipoisoning)	Abdominal pain, nausea, vomiting; anxiety, insomnia, lethargy, headache, musculoskeletal pain and anorexi.
Naproxen (NSAIDs)	Belching, bruising, difficult breathing, headache, itching skin, large, flat, blue, purplish patches in the skin, shortness of breath, skin eruptions and stomach pain.

TABLE 3.2 *Contd...*

Name of Drugs	Adverse Drug Reactions (ADR)
Natamycin (Antiinfective)	Allergic reaction, change in vision, chest pain, corneal opacity, dyspnea, eye discomfort, eye edema, eye hyperemia, eye irritation, eye pain, foreign body sensation, paresthesia, and tearing.
Nefopam (Analgesic, antipyretic)	Nausea, vomiting, sweating, drowsiness, insomnia, urinary retention, dizziness, hypotension, tremor and paraesthesia.
Neomycin (Antibacterial)	Any loss of hearing, clumpsiness, diarrhea, difficulty in breathing, dizziness, drowsiness, decreased frequency urine, increased amount of gas and increased thirst.
Neostigmine (Neuromuscular agent)	Twitches of the muscle visible under the skin, blurred vision, changes speech, chest pain, confusion, cough, difficult breathing, and difficulty in moving.
Netilmicin (Antibacterial)	Headache, malaise, visual disturbances, disorientation, tachycardia, hypotension, palpitations and thrombocytosis.
Nicardipine (Calcium antagonist)	Dizziness, flushing, headache, hypotension, peripheral oedema, tachycardia, palpitations, nausea, dyspepsia and dry mouth.
Nicitinic acid (Anticoagulant)	Darkening of urine, light gray-colored stools, loss of appetite, severe stomach pain, yellow eyes or skin.
Nicotine (Parasympathomimetic)	Headache, cold and flu-like symptoms; insomnia; nausea; myalgia and dizziness; palpitations; dyspepsia and hiccups.
Nicoumalone (Anticoagulant)	Headache altered liver function tests and GI disturbances.
Nifedipine (Antihypertensive)	Bloating or swelling of the face, arms, hands, lower legs, cough, difficult breathing, dizziness,
Nilvadipine (Calcium antagonist)	Headache, peripheral, oedema, dizziness, fatigue, Jaundice, Confusion, Dyspepsia, Anxiety and Chest pain.
Nimodipine (Cardiovascular agent)	Cirrhosis or other liver disease, heart disease, high or low blood pressure.
Nisoldipine (Calcium Channel Blocker)	Dizziness, headache, peripheral oedema, palpitations, pharyngitis, vasodilatation, sinusitis, chest pain and nausea
Nitrazepam (Hypnotic)	Hypotension, palpitation; agitation, aggressiveness, amnesia, ataxia, confusion, delusions, disorientation
Nitrendipine (Antihypertensive)	Hypotension, flushing, oedema, dizziness, palpitation, fatigue, headache, nausea, bloating, diarrhoea
Nitrofurantoin (Antibacterial)	Changes in facial skin colour, chest pain, chills, cough, fever, hives, hoarseness, itching.
Nitroglycerine (Vasodilator)	Bloating or swelling of the face, arms, hands, lower legs, or feet, difficult breathing, feeling faint, dizzy, lightheadedness, feeling of warmth or heat and headache.

TABLE 3.2 Contd...

Name of Drugs	Adverse Drug Reactions (ADR)
Nizatidine (Antiulcer)	Headache and dizziness.
Noradrenaline (Sympathom imetic)	Hypertension, headache, peripheral ischaemia, bradycardia, arrhythmias, anxiety and skin necrosis.
Northiondrone (Hormone)	Menstrual abnormalities, amenorrhea, frequent, irregular, prolonged, or infrequent bleeding, nausea, weight changes, breast changes and headache.
Norethisterone (Gonadal Hormone)	Mental depression, cholestatic jaundice, porphyria, epilepsy, migraine, headache, breast discomfort and dizziness
Norfloxacin (Antibacterial)	Nausea, vomiting, heartburn, constipation, diarrhoea, abdominal cramping, anorexia; headache, dizziness
Nortriptyline (Antidepressant)	Abdominal pain, agitation, anxiety, black, tarry stools, bleeding gums, blood in the urine or stools and blurred vision.
Noscapine (Antitussive, Expectorant)	Loss of coordination, hallucinations , loss of sexual drive, swelling of prostate, loss of appetite, dilated pupils, increased heart rate and chest pains.
Novobiocine (Antibiotic)	Nausea, diarrhoea, vomiting, irritation or soreness of the mouth or rectal area; dyspnoea and eosinophilia.
Nystatin (Antifungal)	Diarrhoea, GI distress, nausea and vomiting. vaginal pessaries/cream: May damage latex contraceptives.
Octretide (Growth Hormone inhibitor)	Gall bladder abnormalities, diarrhea, loose stools, nausea and abdominal discomfort and sinus bradycardia.
Oestradiol (Hormone)	Allergic reaction, difficulty breathing, swelling face, lips, tongue, or throat, vaginal bleeding andchest pain.
Ofloxacin (Antibacterial)	Nausea, vomiting, abdominal pain, diarrhea, headache dizziness, insomnia, hallucination, leucopenia and eosinophilla.
Omeprazole (Proton Pump inhibitor)	Diarrhea, nausea, fatigue, constipation, vomiting, flatulence, acid regurgitation, taste prevention, arthralgia, myalgia, urticaria and dizziness.
Ondansetron (Anti-emetic)	Headache, fatigue, constipation, drowsiness, fever, dizziness, anxiety, cold sensation, pruritus, rash and diarrhea.
Orciprenaline (Antiasthamatic)	Tachycardia, nervousness, increased serum glucose, increased potassium levels, tremor, palpitation and headache.
Ornidazole (Antibacterial)	Somnolence, headache nausea, vomiting, dizziness, tramor, rigidity, poor co coordination, tiredness, vertigo, skin reactions.

TABLE 3.2 Contd...

Name of Drugs	Adverse Drug Reactions (ADR)
Orphenadrine (Antirigidity, antitremor)	Chest pain, chills, cough, fever, hallucinations, headache, shortness of breath, troubled breathing, tightness in chest, skin rash, hives, itching, redness, sores and ulcers mouth.
Oubain (Cardiac glycoside)	Nausea and vomiting pulse irregularities.
Oxacillin (Anitibiotic)	Nausea, vomiting, diarrhea, gastrointestinal irritation, neutropenia, leukopenia, thrombocytopenia, bone marrow depression and hypersensitivity reactions.
Oxamniquine (Anthelmintic)	Allergic reaction, seizures, headache, dizziness, drowsiness, abdominal pain, decreased appetite and vomiting.
Oxaprozin (NSAID)	Skin rash, Bloating, bloody or black, burning upper abdominal pain, cloudy urine, constipation, itching skin, loss of appetite, nausea or vomiting and pale skin.
Oxazepam (Anxiolytic, sedative)	Cyncope, oedema, drowsiness, ataxia, dizziness, vertigo, memory impairment, headache, lethargy, amnesia, rash and euphoria.
Oxprenolol (β-adrenoreceptor antagonist)	Pulmonary oedema, postural hypotension, Prolonged PR interval, sinus arrest, palpitation, chest pain, hot flashes, syncove and vertigo.
Oxybutynin (Anticholinergic)	Dry mouth, constipation, nausea, abdominal pain, blurred vision, headache, dizziness, drowsiness, diarrhea, insomnia.
Oxypentifylline (Muscle pain relaxant)	Nausea, vomiting, dizziness, headache, flushing; angina, palpitations; occasional cardiac arrhythmias and hepatitis.
Oxyphenbutazone (NSAIDs)	Weakness, Headache, Drowsiness, Irritability, Diarrhea, Heart burn, Brushing, Weight loss and Loss of appetite.
Oxytetracycline (Antibacterial)	Anorexia, nausea, vomiting, diarrhea, glssistis, dysphagia, photosensitivity, oesphageal irration & ulceration and nephrotoxicity.
Paclitaxel (Antineoplastic)	Neutropenia, leucopenia, thrombocytopenia, anemia, bleeding, hypersensitivity reactions, bradycardia, abnormal ECG and nausea vomiting.
Pafenolol (Anti hypertension)	Orthostatic hypotension, dizziness, fatigue, vertigo, paraesthesia, headache, nasal stuffiness, dyspnoea and diarrhea.
Pamidronate (Nutritional supplement)	Ocurrence and severity of reactions depend on dose and duration of infusion. Anorexia, dyspepsia, nausea, abdominal pain, vomiting; metastases; fatigue; arthralgia, myalgia; anxiety, headache, insomnia, fever and flu-like symptoms.

TABLE 3.2 *Contd...*

Name of Drugs	Adverse Drug Reactions (ADR)
Pancuronium (Neuromuscular blocker)	Tachycardia, induce miosis, excessive salivation, rashes, itchiness, wheezing, BP increased, cardiac output increased.
Papaverine (Vasodilator)	Allergic reaction, low fever, nausea, stomach pain, loss of appetite, dark urine, clay-colored stools, jaundice, warmth, redness, or tingly feeling in your face, swelling, pain.
Paracetamol (Analgesic, antipyretic)	Nausea, allergic reaction, skin rashes, acute renal tubular necrosis, blood dyscrasias, lever damage.
Paraldehyd (Antiepileptic)	Coughing, skin rash, redness, swelling, pain at injection site, yellow eyes or skin, cloudy urine, confusion, decreased urination, muscle tremors, restlessness and irritability.
Pargyline (MAO-B inhibitor)	Vertigo, Muscle twitching, Blurred vision, Dizziness, Headache, Vomiting, Fever, Insomnia, and Sweating.
Paroxetine (Antidepressant)	Insomnia, headache, dizziness, decreased libido, nausea, xerostomia, constipation, diarrhea, weakness and tramor.
PAS (Antituberculosis)	Abdominal discomfort, fever, skin rashes and nausea.
Pefloxacin (Antibacterial)	Nausea, vomiting gastric pain, dizziness, insomnia, allergic skin reaction, thrombocytopenia, leukopenis and photosensation.
Pelrinone (Misc. Drug)	Headache, tremors, easy bruising or bleeding, chest pain, bronchospasm, low potassium, eadache and tremors.
Pemoline (Monoamine oxidase inhibitor)	Insomnia, nervousness, headache, drowsiness, weight loss, nausea, vomiting and abdominal pain,
Penbutolol (β-adrenoreceptor antagonist)	Headache, dizziness, fatigue, insomnia, asthenia, arrhythmia, diaphoresis, CHF, nausea, diarrhoea, dyspepsia, upper resp tract infection, dyspnoea, cough, chest and limb pain, excessive sweating and impotence.
Penicillamine (Antigout)	Nausea, anorexia, vomiting, oral ulceration, stomatitis, fever and skin reaction, lass of test, thrombocytopenia and neutropenis.
Pentaerythritoltn (Antianginal)	Cardiovascular: Flushing, postural hypotension, headache, lightheadedness, dizziness, neuromuscular & skeletal weakness, Drug rash and exfoliative dermatitis.
Pentamidine (Antimicrobial)	Headache, disorientation, hallucinations, dizziness, confusion, fatigue, neuralgia, chest pain, ECG abnormalities, syncope, vasodilation, vasculitis, phlebitis, hypertension, palpitations, arrhythmias, severe hypotension and pharyngitis.
Pentazocine (Analgesic, antipyretic)	Physical dependence, sedation, dizziness, euphoria, alteration of mood, respiratory depression, visual hallucination and disorientation and confusion.

TABLE 3.2 Contd...

Name of Drugs	Adverse Drug Reactions (ADR)
Pentobarbitone (Sedative)	Residual sedation, drowsiness, lethargy, vertigo, nausea, vomiting, headache, Behavioral problems, impaired memory, tics, dyskinesias and nystagmus.
Pentoxifylline (Peripheral vasodilator)	Nausea, vomiting, dizziness, headache, flushing, angina, palpitation, jaundice, blood dyscrasias reported, agitation and sleep disturbances.
Pergolide (Anti parkinson's disease)	Anxiety, bloody or cloudy urine, confusion, difficult or painful urination, frequent urge to urinate, hallucinations uncontrolled movements of the body,
Pencyazine (Antipsychotic)	Drowsiness, dizziness, dries mouth, nausea, vomiting, constipation, diarrhea, uncontrolled muscle movements, patches on skin, weight gain, decreased libido.
Permdopril (Anti hypertensive)	Renal dysfunction, pancreatitis, blood disorders (e.g. agranulocytosis, neutropenia, thrombocytopenia). Cough, dizziness, vertigo, hypotension, headache, asthenia, back pain, sinusitis, chest pain, abnormal ECG, sleep disorders, viral infection, upper extremity pain, hypertonia, fever, proteinuria, ear infection, palpitation, GI disorders (e.g. nausea, dyspepsia, abdominal pain) and rash.
Perphenazine (Antipsychotic)	Hanges in BP, orthostatic hypotension, changes in heart rate, dizziness; extrapyramidal symptoms and dizziness.
Pethidine (Analgesic)	Hypotension; fatigue, drowsiness, dizziness, nervousness and headache.
Phenethecilline (Semi synthetic penicillin)	Nausea, vomiting, dizziness, headache, flushing; angina, palpitations; occasional cardiac arrhythmias and hepatitis.
Phenelzine (MOA inhibitor)	Dizziness, dry mouth, headache, lethargy, sedation, insomnia, anorexia, weight gain, nausea, vomiting, diarrhea, tramour, hyperthermia and sweting.
Phenformin (Oral antidiabetic)	Metallic taste, wt loss, skin reactions, acute pancreatitis, Lactic acidosis and CV adverse effects
Phenindamine (Respiratory agent)	Drowsiness, dizziness, headache, loss of appetite, stomach upset, visual disturbances, irritability, dry mouth. CNS stimulation may occur in certain individuals.
Phenindione (Anticoagulant)	Hypersensitivity reactions e.g. exfoliative dermatitis, liver and kidney damage, myocarditis, agranulocytosis, leucopenia, eosinophilia and leukaemoid syndrome.
Pheniramine (Antiallergics)	Oral sedation, hypersensitivity reaction, lassitude, dizziness, tinnitus, inability to concentrate, incoordination, irritability, insomnia and trammors.
Phenobarbitone (Anticonvulsant)	Brabycardia, hypotension, drowsiness, lethargy, CNS excitation or depression, impaired judgment and hangover effect.

TABLE 3.2 *Contd...*

Name of Drugs	Adverse Drug Reactions (ADR)
Phenoxy-Mepenicillin (Antibiotic)	Nasal congestion, slight GI irritation, miosis, postural hypotension with dizziness, fatigue.
Phentermine (Monoamine oxidase inhibitor)	Urticaria, GI upsets palpitations, tachycardia, elevated blood pressure, overstimulation, restlessness, insomnia, tremor, headache, dry mouth, dizziness, dysphoria, euphoria, psychosis, changes in libido and impotence.
Phenylbutazone (Antiinflammatory)	Tachycardia, hypotension, myocarditis, atrial fibrillation, atrial flutter, angina, CHF, myocardial depression.
Phenylethyl-malonamide (Anticonvulsant)	Drowsiness, ataxia; nausea, vomiting and hepatic.
Phenylephrine (Mydriatic / cycloplegic)	Anxiety, reflex bradycardia, tachycardia, arrhythmias, headache, cold extrimetis, hypertension, nausea, vomiting, fever, weakness and sweting.
Phenyl propanolamine (Stimulant, Decongestant)	Hypertension, epileptic seizures, hallucinations, dizziness, headache, nausea and palpitation.
Phenytoin (Antiarrythmatic)	Hypersensitivity, lack of appetite, headache, dizziness, tremor, insomnia, GI disturbances, acne and hirsutism.
Pholcodine (Respiratory agent)	Dizziness, occasional drowsiness, nausea, vomiting, constipation, rash, sputum retention, excitation and confusion,
Physostigmine (Parasympathomimetic)	Heart failure, high or low blood pressure, ever had a heart attack, asthma, a stomach ulcer or stomach spasms, Epilepsy, hyperthyroidism and Parkinson's disease.
Pimozide (Antipsychotic)	Extra pyramidal reaction, insomnia, drowsiness, dizziness, ECG changes, dry mouth, constipation and urinary difficulty.
Pinacidil (Antihypertensive)	Tachycardia, palpitation, edema, dizziness, headache, nausea, palpitation, tachycardia, rashes, increased intracranial pressure.
Pindolol (β-adrenoreceptor antagonist)	Bradycardia, hypotension, peripheral oedema, heart failure, bronco spasm, fatigue, dizziness, insomnia and dizzarre dreams.
Pipecuronium (Neuromuscular Blocker)	Anaphylactic reactions and malignant hyperthermia.
Piperacillin (β-lactam antibiotic)	GI disturbances, hypersensitivity reactions, eosinophillia, hyponatraemia, pypokalaemia, injection site related reaction like painerythema and induration.
Piperazine (Anthelmintic)	Nausea, vomiting, colic, abdominal pain, diarrhea, urticaria, skin rashes, headache, bronchospasm, dizziness and mystagmus.

TABLE 3.2 Contd...

Name of Drugs	Adverse Drug Reactions (ADR)
Pipothiazine (Typical antipsychotic)	Dyskinesia, leucopenia, agranulocytosis, hypothermia, leucocytosis, cardiovascular symptoms, extrapyramidal effects and haemolytic anemia.
Piracetam (Neurotransmitter gamma-aminobutyric acid)	Hyperkinesia, nervousness, depression, diarrhoea, rashes. CNS stimulation, sleep disturbances and dizziness.
Pipothiazine (Antipsychotic)	Parkinsonian symptoms, dystonia, akathisia, tardive dyskinesia and Interference with temp regulation.
Piracetam (Nootropic Drug)	Hyperkinesia, nervousness, depression, diarrhoea, rashes. CNS stimulation, sleep disturbances and dizziness.
Pirbuterol (Cerebral activator)	Headache, dizziness, lightheadedness, insomnia, tremor or nervousness, sweating, nausea, vomiting, or diarrhea, or dry mouth and allergic reaction.
Pirenzepine (Anti-ulcer drug)	Dry mouth, blurred vision, drowsiness, dizziness, nausea, heartburn, diarrhea, constipation, bitter taste, decreased sexual ability or desire and bad breath.
Piretanide (Loop diuretic)	Thrombocytopenia, ototoxicity, hypotension, dehydration, leucopenia, hyponatremia, urinary retention, gout, cardiac arrhythmia, renal failure and hypotension.
Piroxicam (NSAIDs)	GI disturbances, peptic ulcer, GI bleeding, headache, dizziness, blurred vision, tinnitus, skin rashes and pruritus.
Pirprofen (Antiinflammatory)	GI disturbances, peptic ulcer, headache, dizziness, blurred vision, tinnitus, skin rashes and pruritus.
Pivampicillin (Antibiotic)	Hypersensitivity reactions including urticaria; fever; joint pains; rashes; angioedema; serum sickness-like reactions.
Pivmecillinam (Antibiotic)	Hypersensitivity reactions including uticaria; fever; joint pains; rashes; angioedema; serum sickness-like reactions and gastrointestinal disturbances.
Pizotifen (Analgesic)	Sedation, dry mouth, drowsiness, increased appetite and weight gain. CNS depression; headache, psychomotor impairment, antimuscarinic effects and GI disturbances.
Polymixin B (Antibacterial)	Dizziness, paraesthesia, muscle weakens, atexia, confusion, drowsiness, psuchoses, convulsion, coma and neuromuscular block.
Polythiazide (Diuretic)	Abdominal or stomach pain, black, tarry stools, bleeding, gums, bloating, blood in urine or stools,
Practolol (β-adrenorceptor/ antagonist)	Bronchoconstriction, cardiac failure, cold extremities, fatigue and depression, hypoglycaemia, oculomuco-cutaneous syndrome.

TABLE 3.2 Contd...

Name of Drugs	Adverse Drug Reactions (ADR)
Pravastatin (Anti-cholesterol)	GI symptoms, headache, insomnia, chest pain, rash, fatigue, dizziness, myalgia, hypersensitivity, anaphylaxis and angioedema.
Prazepam (Hypnotic)	Drowsiness, sedation, muscle weakness and ataxia; less frequently vertigo, headache, confusion and depression.
Praziquantel (Anthelmintic)	Headache, drowsiness, dizziness, malasia, abdominal discomfort, nausea vomiting, diarrhea, rashes and urticaria.
Prazosin (Antihypertensive)	Postural hypotension, syncope, palpitation, lack of energy, nausea, oedema, chest pain, dyspnoea, constipation and vomiting.
Prednisolone (Cortico steroid)	Cushing's syndrome, & growth, retardation in childn; osteoporosis, fractures, peptic ulceration; glaucoma cataracts, hyperglycemia, pancreatitis.
Prednisone (Cortico steroid)	Insomnia, nervousness, increased appetite, indigestion, dizziness, headache and hirsutism
Prenalterol (Cerebral vasodialator)	Bronchospasm, peripheral vasospasm, constipation and diarrhea.
Prenyleamine (Calcium channel blocker)	Liver damage and parkinson's disease.
Primaquine (Antimalarial)	Nausea, vomiting, epigastria distress, abdominal cramps, leucopenia, leucocytosis, agranulocytosis, haemolytic anemia and thrombocytopaenia.
Primidone (Anticonvulsant)	Drowsiness, ataxia, nausea, vomiting, visual disturbances, rashes, nystagmus, vertigo and hypersensitivity.
Prilocaine (Local Anesthetic)	Methemoglobinaemia; cyanosis, restlessness, excitement, nervousness, paraesthesias, dizziness, tinnitus and blurred vision.
Probenecid (Antigout drug)	Mild nausea, vomiting, stomach pain, loss of appetite, headache, dizziness, hair loss, warmth or tingly feeling.
Procaine (Local anaesthetic)	GI upsets; diarrhoea; flatulence; abdominal pain; nausea; vomiting and Hypersensitivity reactions.
Procarbazine (Antincoplastic)	Severe hypotension, ventricular fibrillation and asystole with rapid IV admin. Drug-induced SLE syndrome.
Prochlorperazine (Antiemetic, antinauseants)	Allergic reaction, chest pain or slow or irregular heartbeats, dizziness, drowsiness, anxiety, nausea or vomiting and seizures.
Procyclidine (Antirigidity, antitremor)	GI disturbances, anorexia, nausea and vomiting; bone marrow depression; leukopenia and thrombocytopaenia.
Progabide (Antiepileptic)	Cholestatic jaundice, cardiac arrhythmia, orthostatic hypotension, leucopaneia, thrombocytopaenis, dry mouth, blurring of vision and glaucoma.

TABLE 3.2 Contd...

Name of Drugs	Adverse Drug Reactions (ADR)
Progesterone (Gonadal Hormone)	Excitability, dizziness, hallucination, dry mouth, blurred vision, constipation, urinary retention, agitation and confusion.
Proguanil (Antimalarial)	GI disturbances, headache, vertigo, rash, haematological abnormality in persons with renal impairment and dermatological reactions.
Promazine (Antipsychotic)	GI disturbance, appetite, fluid retension, oedema, acne, skin rash, urticaria, depression, headache, fever and fatigue.
Promethazine (Anti emetic, antin-auseants)	Nausea, vomiting, abdominal pain, headache, diarrhea, weakness, loss of appetite, and dizziness, fever and mouth sores.
Propafenone (Antiarrythmatic)	Drowsiness, dystonia, akathisia, dyskinesia, Fever, altered consciousness, autonomic dysfunction, insomnia, nausea, vomiting and constipation.
Propantheline (Prokinetics)	CNS depressions, paradoxical excitation in childn, dryness of mouth, blurring of ision, retension of urine, constipation and trachucardia.
Propofol (Anaesthetics)	Dizziness, visual disturbances, vertigo dry mouth, headache, GI disturbances, alternation in test, allergic skin and rashes.
Propranolol (β-blocker)	Dry mouth, thrust, difficulty in swallowing, skin dryness, flashing, reduced sweating, heat stroke, constipation and nausea.
Propylthiouracil (Thyroid agent)	Involuntary muscle movements, nausea, vomiting, headache, fever, pain, burning or stinging at injection site and apnoea.
Protriptyline (Antidepressant)	Transient hypertension, hypertension, dizziness, flashing, fatigue, drowsiness, weakness, seizures, nausea and vomiting.
Pyrantel (Anthelmintic)	Black, tarry stools, chest pain, chills, cough, fever, painful or difficult urination, shortness of breath, sore throat, sores, ulcers, or white spots on the lips or in the mouth.
Pyrazinamide (Antituberculers)	Myocardial infarction, stroke, heart block, arrhythmias, particularly orthostatic hypotension and hypertension.
Pyridostigmine (Misc. agent)	Muscarinic side effects e.g. nausea, vomiting, diarrhoea, abdominal cramps, increased peristalsis, increased salivation, increased bronchial secretions, miosis and diaphoresis. Nicotinic side effects include muscle cramps, fasciculation and weakness.
Pyrimethamine (Antiprotozoal)	Fever, irritation or soreness of tongue, skin rash, black, tarry stools, bleeding or crusting sores on lips, blood in urine or stools, chest pain and chills.

TABLE 3.2 Contd...

Name of Drugs	Adverse Drug Reactions (ADR)
Quazepam (Hypnotic)	Drowsiness, dizziness, anxiety, dry mouth, hyperventilation, increased muscle spasm, irregular heartbeats, irritability, nervousness, nightmares and restlessness.
Quinacrine (Anthelmintic)	Abdominal pain, stomach cramps, diarrhea, fever, headache, loss of appetite, pelvic pain, vaginal itching, nausea and vomiting.
Quinalbarbitone (Barbiturate)	Somnolence, Impaired motor functions, Impaired coordination, Impaired balance, Dizziness, Anxiety, Confusion, Agitation, irritability, or excitability and Headache
Quinidine (Antiarrythmic)	Diarrhea, loss of appetite, muscle weakness, nausea or vomiting, abdominal pain and/or yellow eyes and confusion.
Quinine (Antimalarial)	Muscle weakness, nausea vomiting, diarrhea, cinchonism symptoms including impaired hearing, headache, blurred vision, dizziness, vomiting.
Quinapril (Antihypertensive)	Cough dizziness, fatigue, nausea, vomiting, hypotension, allergic reaction, feeling light-headed, fainting, fever, chills, body aches and flu symptoms.
Ramipril (Antihypertensive)	Nausea, vomiting, diarrhea, dizziness, fatigue, headache, abdominal pain and cough.
Ranitidine (H_2 receptor antagonist)	Headache, malaise, dizziness, somnolence, insomnia, vertigo, reversible mental confusion, agitation, mental depression, hallucinations, constipation, nausea, vomiting, abdominal discomfort or pain, rash (urticaria, maculopapular, and/or pruritic), loss of libido. Small increases in serum creatinine.
Reproterol (Respiratory agent)	Fine tremor of skeletal muscle, palpitations, muscle cramps, tachycardia, nervous tension and headache.
Reserpine (Antihypertensive)	Nasal congestion, headache, CNS disorders, Gi disturbance, Brest engorgement, galactorrhoea, gynaecomastia, decreased libido.
Ribavirin (Antiviral)	Increased serum bilirubin and uric acid, haemolytic anemia, reticulocytosis, anorexia, dyspepsia, nausea, vomiting and irritability.
Rifabutine (Antibiotic)	Diarrhea, fever, heartburn, indigestion, loss of appetite, nausea, skin itching and rash.
Rifampicin (Antitubarcular)	GI disturbances, pseudomembranous colitis, abnormalities of liver function, liver disorders, influenza like symptoms and skin reactions.

TABLE 3.2 *Contd...*

Name of Drugs	Adverse Drug Reactions (ADR)
Rimantadine (Antiviral)	Nausea, vomiting, abdominal pain, diarrhoea, dyspepsia, xerostomia, taste alteration, anorexia and headache.
Rimiterol (Respiratory agent)	Fine tremor of skeletal muscle, palpitations, muscle cramps, tachycardia, nervous tension and headache.
Risperidone (Antipsychotic)	Agitation, anxiety, dizziness, headache, somnolence, orthostatic hypotension, constipation, dyepepsia, nausea and vomiting.
Roxatidine (Antihyperacidic agent)	Occasional headache, GI disturbances, gynaecomastia, alopecia, blood dyscrasias, pancreatitis, sleep disturbances, restlessness and dizziness.
Roxithromycin (Antibacterial)	Nausea, vomiting, abdominal pain, diarrhea, weakness, malaise, anorexia, constipation, dyspepsia, hepatitis and rashes.
Salbutamol (Antiasthamic)	Fine skeletal muscle tremor especially hands, tachycardia, palpitations, muscle cramps, headache, paradoxical bronchospasm, angioedema, urticaria, hypotension and collapse.
Salicylate (Analgesic)	GI disorders, fatigue, hypersensitivity reactions, skin eruptions, haemolytic anaemia, weakness and dyspnoea.
Salsalate (Antiinflammatory)	GI symptoms, hypersensitivity reactions, skin eruptions, angioedema, weakness, rhinitis and dyspnoea.
Scopolamine (Anti-acetylcholine)	Dry mouth, dyshidrosis, tachycardia, bradycardia, urinary retention, hallucinations and agitation.
Secbutobarbitone (Barbiturate)	Drowsiness, ataxia, paradoxical excitement, confusion, headache and CNS depression; respiratory depression; GI disorders; hepatitis: fever; megaloblastic anaemia.
Secobarbital (Hypnotic)	Unwanted sleepiness, trouble waking up, dizziness, excitation, headache, tiredness, loss of appetite, nausea and vomiting.
Selegiline (Antirigidity & antitremor)	Hallucination, dizziness, confusion, anxiety, dreams, palpitations, syncope, irritability, restlessness, nausea, vomiting and dry mouth.
Semustine (Antincoplastic)	Bone marrow suppression, stomach ache, hemorrhagic cystitis, diarrhea, darkening of the skin, alopecia, changes in color and texture of the hair, and lethargy.
Sertraline (Antidepressant)	Nausea, vomiting, anorexia, dyspepsia, constipation, diarhoea, dry mouth, vomiting, ejaculation failure, increased sweating.
Simvastatin (Lipid lowering agent)	Headache, nausea, flatulence, heartburn, abdominal pain, diarrhea, dysgeusia and hypensensitivity.

TABLE 3.2 Contd...

Name of Drugs	Adverse Drug Reactions (ADR)
Succinylsulfathiazole (Anti Microbial)	Allergic reactions, vomiting and diarrhea.
Sodium cromoglycate (Antiasthmatic)	Nausea, headache, dizziness, unpleasant taste, joint pain and swelling, skin rashes, aggrevation of asthma and pulmonary inflitates.
Sotalol (Antihypertensive)	Fatigue, vertigo, dyspnea, bradycardia, headaches, occasionally edema, nausea, diarrhea and hypotension.
Spectinomycin (Antibacterial)	Dizziness; nausea; urticaria; chills; fever; headache, insomnia, mild to moderate pain after injection.
Spironolactone (Antidiuretic)	Numbness or tingly feeling, muscle pain or weakness, slow, fast, or uneven heart rate, feeling drowsy, restless, shallow breathing, tremors, confusion.
Streptokinase (Anticoagulant)	Fever, chills, back pain, abdominal pain, nausea, vomiting, arthythmia, brushing, rash, pruritus and allergic reaction.
Streptomycin (Antibacterial)	Giddiness, vertigo, tinnitus, atexia, hypersensitivity reaction, ototoxicity & nephrodoxicity, anaphylactic shock, aplastic anemia and agranulocytosis.
Streptozocin (Antineoplastic)	Swelling of feet or lower legs, unusual decrease in urination, Nausea and vomiting, anxiety, nervousness, chills, cold sweats and pale skin.
Sufentanil (Anaesthetic)	GI disturbances. Difficulty with micturition, ureteric or biliary spasm; dry mouth; sweating; headache and facial flushing.
Sulfadiazine (Anti Microbial)	Nausea, vomiting, anorexia, diarrhea, hypersensitivity, skin reaction, lumber pain, haematoria, olguria, anuria and cryslatization in urine.
Sulfadimethoxine (Anti Microbial)	Anemia, lethargic, vomiting, loss of appetite, joint pain and kidney damage.
Sulfafurazole (Anti Microbial)	Nausea, vomiting, anorexia, diarrhoea, hypersensitivity reactions, SLE, serum sickness-like syndrome.
Sulfamethiazole (Anti Microbial)	Nausea, vomiting, anorexia, diarrhoea, hypersensitivity reactions, blood disorders, serum sickness-like syndrome.
Sulfamethoxy-pyridazine (Anti Microbial)	Dizziness or vertigo; acute renal failure, interstitial nephritis, acute tubular necrosis and electrolyte imbalances.
Sulfamethoxazole (Anti Microbial)	Loss of appetite, nausea, vomiting, bleeding, aplastic anemia, jaundice, hepatic necrosis, mouth sores, joint aches, severe skin rashes and itching.
Sulfametopyrazine (Antibacterial)	Nausea, vomiting, anorexia, diarrhoea, hypersensitivity reactions, SLE, serum sickness-like syndrome, liver necrosis and hepatomegaly, myocarditis, pulmonary eosinophilia and fibrosing alveolitis, vasculitis, hypoglycaemia, hypothyroidism, neurological reactions, jaundice and kernicterus in premature neonates and Pseudomembranous colitis.

TABLE 3.2 Contd...

Name of Drugs	Adverse Drug Reactions (ADR)
Sulfasalazine (Anti Microbial)	Headache, anorexia, nausea, vomiting, diarrhea, abdominal discomfort, photosensitivity, crystalluria, slaining of contact lens and alopecia.
Sulfathiazole (Anti Microbial)	Localized irritation, allergy and Stevens-Johnson syndrome
Sulfaurea (Antibacterial)	Irritation, stinging, burning of the skin, allergic reactions, bloody diarrhea, fever, joint pain, red and swollen.
Sulfinopyrazone (Antigout)	Nausea, vomitting, diarrhoea, skin rashes, renal impairment or failure, salt and water retention and blood dyscrasia.
Sulfisoxazole (Sulphonamide antibacterial)	Anxiety, blurred vision, changes in menstrual periods, chills, cold sweats, coma, and confusion, cool and pale skin.
Sulindac (Antiinflammatory)	Acid or sour stomach, belching, constipation, headache, heartburn, nausea or vomiting, skin rash and stomach pain.
Sulipride (Antipsychotic)	Postural hypotension, hyperprolactinaemia, weight gain, sedation, insomnia and extrapyramidal symptoms.
Sulphadiamidine (Antibacterial)	Nausea, vomiting, anorexia, diarrhoea, hypersensitivity reactions, SLE and serum sickness-like syndrome
Sulphadiazine (Antibacterial)	Rash, fainting, blood in the urine, difficult or painful urination, yellowing of the skin or eyes, ringing in the ears, difficulty breathing, sore throat, chills and skin rash.
Sulphadoxine (Antiprotozole)	Fever, increased sensitivity of skin to sunlight, irritation or soreness of tongue, skin rash, Black, tarry stools and chest pain.
Sulphaguanidine (Antibacterial)	GI effects, hypersensitivity reactions, nephrotoxic reactions, CV effects, hypoglycaemia, hypothyroidism and neurological reactions.
Sulphamethoxazole (Antibacterial)	Loss of appetite, nausea, vomiting. Patient's allergic, bleeding, aplastic anemia, jaundice, hepatic necrosis, mouth sores, joint aches, severe skin rashes and itching.
Sulphasazine (antigout)	Aching of joints, fever, and headache, increased sensitivity of the skin to sunlight, skin rash, and itching, vomiting, back, leg and stomach pains.
Sulphinpyrazone (Antigout)	Nausea, vomitting, diarrhoea, skin rashes, renal impairment or failure, salt and water retention and blood dyscrasia.
Sumatriptan (Antimigrain)	Transient hypertension, hypotension, dizziness, flashing, fatigue, drowsiness, weakness, seizures, nausea, vomiting and parasethesia.
Sutamicillin (Antibiotic)	Diarrhoea, nausea, vomitting, rashes, pruritus, blood dyscrasias, superinfections, dizziness and dyspnoea.
Tacrine (Parasympathomimetic)	Dizziness, headache, nausea, vomiting, diarrhoea, myalgia and ataxia.

TABLE 3.2 *Contd...*

Name of Drugs	Adverse Drug Reactions (ADR)
Tacrolimus (Immunosuppressive drug)	Tremor, headache, paraesthesias, nausea, vomiting, diarrhea, hypertension, blood dyscrasias, leucocytosis, inpaired ranal function.
Talampicillin (Antibiotic)	Diarrhea, allergic reactions, severe stomach pain, unusual bruising or bleeding and jaundice.
Tamoxifen (Antineoplastic)	Hot flashes, oedema, fluid retension, dry skin, vaginal bleeding, vaginal discharge, pruritus valve, GI upsets, nausea, vomiting.
Temazepam (Anxiolytic)	CNS depression, somnolence, dizziness, fatigue, ataxia, lethargy, impairment of memory and learning and reduced alertness.
Teniposide (Chemotherapeutic agent)	Reversible alopoecia, nausea, vomiting, diarrhoea, mucositis, rash, fever, neurotoxicity, hepatic or renal problem.
Tenoxicam (NSAIDs)	GI upset including epigastric pain & gastritis, nausea, vomiting, hypersensitivity reaction, headache, dizziness and sleep disturbances.
Terazocin (Antihypertensive)	Orthoseaeic hypotension, syncope, dizziness, fatigue, somnolence, peripheral oedema, headache and nasal congestion.
Terbutaline (Bronchodilator)	Fine skeletal muscle tremor especially hands, flashes, dizziness, anxiety, swelling, nausea, vomiting, lethargy, tinnitus and trachycardia.
Terconezole (Antifungal drug)	Asthenia, fever, chills, nausea, vomiting, myalgia, arthralgia, malaise, hypersensitivity, anaphylaxis, face edema, dizziness, bronchospasm and skin rash.
Terfenadine (Antihistamine)	Drowsiness or dizziness, headache, nervousness, nausea, diarrhea, abdominal discomfort, dry mouth and dry skin or itchiness.
Testosterone (Gonadal Hormone)	Fluid & electrolyte reaction, increased vascularity of skin, hypercalcemia, impaired glucose toleracce and increased bone growth.
Tetrabenzine (Antirigidity & Antitremor)	Body aches, pain, chills, cough, difficulty in breathing, difficulty with swallowing, discouragement, drowsiness, ear congestion, fear or nervousness and fever and irritability.
Tetracycline (Antibiotic)	Oesophageal ulceration, nausea, vomiting, oral candidiasis, diarrhea, epigasteic burning, sore throat and black hairy tongue and pancreatitis.
Tetrayhdroca-nnabinol (Hallucinogen)	Photosensitivity reaction, dry mouth, hepatitis, thrombocytopenia, generalized edema and depression and pruritus.

TABLE 3.2 Contd...

Name of Drugs	Adverse Drug Reactions (ADR)
Thalidomide (Leprosy, cancer)	Severe and irreversible peripheral neuropathy, constipation dizziness, orthostatic hypotension and drowsiness.
Theobromine (Vasodilator)	Nausea, vomiting, dizziness, headache and flushing.
Theophylline (Bronchodilator)	Nausea, vomiting, abdominal pain, headache, diarrhea, insomnia, dizziness, anxiety, restlessness and tremor.
Thiabendazole (Anthelmintic)	Confusion, diarrhea, hallucinations, irritability, loss of appetite, nausea, vomiting, numbness or tingling in the hands or feet.
Thramphenicol (Antibiotic)	Hypersensitivity, GI disturbances, stomatitis, glossitis, encephalopathy, mental depression and headache.
Thioguanine (Antineoplastic)	Black, tarry stools, blood in urine or stools, cough or hoarseness, fever, chills, lower back or side pain, painful or difficult urination, pinpoint red spots on skin.
Thiopental (Sedative)	Coughing, hiccupping, sneezing, muscle twitching, laryngospasm, bronchospasm, tissue necrosis and burning pain.
Thioridazine (Antipsychotic)	Drowsiness, dry mouth, blurred vision, dizziness, sedation, antimuscarinic affects postural hypotension and akathisia.
Thiotepa (Antineoplastic)	GI disturbances; fatigue, weakness, headache and dizziness; hypersensitivity reactions; blurred vision and conjunctivitis; amenorrhoea, impaired fertility; local irritation, frank chemical or haemorrhagic cystitis; depigmentation of periorbital skin (eye drops).
Thymoxamine (Calcium antagonist)	Nausea; diarrhoea; flushing; headache; dizziness; dry mouth; nasal congestion and hepatotoxicity.
Thyroxine (Thyroidal Hormone)	Chest pain or discomfort, decreased urine output, difficult or labored breathing, difficulty with swallowing, dilated neck veins, extreme fatigue, fainting and fever.
Tiapamil (Calcium antagonist)	CNS disturbances, dizziness; visual disturbances (blurred or yellowish vision) and arrhythmia
Tiaprofenic acid (Antiinflammatory)	Drowsiness, dizziness, headache, stomach upset, nausea, diarrhea, trouble sleeping, irritability, constipation and dry mouth.
Ticarcillin (Antibiotic)	Hypersensitivity reactions, GI disturbances, pseudo-membranous colitis and blood dyscrasias,
Ticlopidine (Anticoagulant)	Diarrhea, nausea, dyspepsia, bleeding pupura, skin rash, increase in serum cholesterol concentration and hepatitis.
Timolol (Antiglucoma)	Fatigue, headache, coldness of extremist, paraesthesia, GI synptoms, Dyspnoea, Skin rash, alopecia, dry mouth, bradicardia.

TABLE 3.2 Contd...

Name of Drugs	Adverse Drug Reactions (ADR)
Tinidazole (Antibacterial)	Metallic taste, nausea, headache, vomiting, dark urine, flushing, anorexia, diarrhea, tiredness, transient leucopenis.
Tobramycin (Antibacterial)	Nausea, vomiting, dizziness, acute renal failure, intestinal nephritis, acute tubular necrosis, electrolyte inbalances and purpura.
Tocainide (Antiarrythmic)	Dizziness, lightheadedness, loss of appetite, nausea, blurred vision, confusion, headache and nervousness.
Tolazoline (Vasodilator)	Piloerection, headache, flushing, nausea, vomiting, diarrhoea, epigastric pain, tachycardia and cardiac arrhythmias.
Tolazamide (Antidiabetic)	Abdominal, stomach pain, chills, clay colored stools, dark urine, diarrhea, difficulty swallowing and dizziness.
Tolbutamide (Hypoglycemic Drug)	Hypoglycemia, nausea, vomiting, epigastric fullness, heartburn, headache, allergic skin reactions and jaundice.
Tolfenamic acid (NSAIDS)	Dysuria especially in males; diarrhoea, nausea, epigastric pain, vomiting, dyspepsia, erythema, headache. Tremor, euphoria, fatigue and pulmonary infiltration.
Tolmetin (Antiinflammatory)	Nausea, dyspepsia, diarrhoea, flatuence, vomiting, headache, GI bleed, hypersensitivity reactions and asthenia.
Tolrestat (Antidiabetic)	Hepatotoxicity and heart valve disorder.
Torsemide (Diuretic)	Electrolyte disturbances, hypokalemia, dehydration, dry mouth, headache, dizziness, hypotension, weakness, drowsiness, and confessional states.
Tranexamic acid (Anti Fibinolic)	Diarrhea, nausea, vomiting, disturbance in colour vision, giddiness and hypertension.
Tranylcypromine (MOA inhibitor)	Absence of or decrease in body movement, actions that are out of control, agitation, anxiety, black, tarry stools, bleeding gums, blood in the urine or stools and chest pain.
Trazodone (Antidepressant)	Drowsiness, dizziness, restlessness, confusional state, headache, nausea, vomiting, weakness, weight loss, dry mouth, constipation, diarrhoea, tremor, bradycardia or tachycardia, orthostatic hypotension, oedema, blurred vision, priapism, skin rash, syndrome of inappropriate secretion of antidiuretic hormone.
Triamcinolone (Cortecosteroid)	Allergic reactions, certain types of arthritis, gout and skin diseases.
Triamterene (Cardiovascular agent)	Photosensitivity reactions, increase in uric acid concentrations, megaloblastic anemia, thrombocytopenia and hyperkalaemia.
Triancinolone (Corticosteroid)	HPA exis suppression, intracranial hypertension, cushings syndrome, growth reduction in children, osterprosis and feactures.

TABLE 3.2 Contd...

Name of Drugs	Adverse Drug Reactions (ADR)
Triazolam (Anxiolytic)	Somnolence, dizziness, feeling of lightness, coordination problems, tachycardia, tiredness, confusional states, memory impairment, cramps and depression.
Trichloro ethanol (Sedative-hypnotic)	Gastric irritation, abdominal distention and flatulence
Trifluoperazine (Anti Psychotic)	Heart disease high blood pressure, angina, severe asthma, emphysema, glaucoma, seizures, pheochromocytoma, Parkinson's disease, hypocalcemia.
Trimeprazine (Respiratory agent)	Hypoglycemia, Depression, Hypotension, Tachycardia, Respiratory failure, Hypoventilation.
Trimethoprim (Anti Bacterial)	Abdominal, stomach pain, black, tarry stools, blistering, peeling, or loosening of the skin, changes in skin color, chest pain, chills, cough or hoarseness and dizziness.
Trimipramine (Antidepressant)	Dry mouth, accommodation disturbances, tachycardia, and constipation, hesitancy of micturation, drowsiness, sweating, postural hypotension, skin rashes, cholestatic jaundice, hypomania, convulsions, cardiac arrhythmias and peripheral neuropathy. Agitation and confusion (elderly).
Tripolidine (Respiratory agent)	CNS depression, headache, psychomotor impairment, dry mouth, thickened respiratory tract secrations, blurred vision, urinary difficulty or retension.
Tubocurarine (Neuromuscular blocker)	Anaphylactoid reactions, apnea, cardiovascular collapse, ganglionic blockage, postoperative respiratory failure, urticaria and erythema.
Urapidil (Antihypertensive)	Dizziness, nausea, headache, fatigue, orthostatic hypotension and palpitations.
Valproate (Antiepileptic)	Asthenia, nausea, diarrhea, abdominal pain, thrombocytopenia, weight gain, peripheral edema, tremor, insomnia.
Vancomycin (Antibacterial)	Otoloxicity, nephrotoxicity, eosinophilla, urticaria, thrombopholoebitis, tryeresensivity reacns, Stevens Johnson syndrome.
Vecuronium (Neuromuscular blocker)	Muscle weakness, paralysis, muscle atrophy, hypersensitivity reactions, ulticiria & aerythema, anaphylaxis and respiratory failure.
Venlafaxine (Anti-depressant)	Nausea, vomiting, anorexia, dry mouth constipation, orthostatic hypotension, tramor, sweating, rash, anxiety, dizziness and fatigue.
Verapamil (Antihypertensive)	Bradicardia, CHF, MI, AV block, worsening heart failure, transient asystole, hypotension, pulmonary edema, nausea and fatigue.
Vidarabine (Antiviral)	Irritation; pain; superficial punctate keratitis; photophobia; lachrymation; blockage of lachrymal duct and temporary visual haze.

TABLE 3.2 *Contd...*

Name of Drugs	Adverse Drug Reactions (ADR)
Vigabatrin (Antiepileptic)	Drowsiness, fatigue, dizziness, nervousness, irritability, headache, confusion, depression, aggression, psychosis, excitation and agitation in child, memory disturbance, irreversible visual field defects, diplopia, weight gain, GI disturbances, ataxia, paraesthesia, tremor, inability to concentrate, hepatitis and Decreased LFT and haemoglobin.
Viloxazine (Antidepressant)	Headache, nausea, vomiting, drowsiness, tremor, ataxia, antimuscarinic side effects (e.g. dry mouth, constipation); musculoskeletal pain; mild hypertension; skin rashes; convulsions; jaundice and increase in LFT.
Vinblastin (Anticancer)	Increased toxicity of vinblastine with erythromycin. Increased neurotoxicity and myelotoxicity with azole antifungals e.g. itraconazole and posaconazole. Increased risk of severe neutropenia with ritonavir. Increased risk of acute pulmonary toxicity with mitomycin. Increased toxicity when ganciclovir is given with, immediately before or after vinblastine.
Vincristine (Anti Cancer)	Hyperuricaemia, bronchospasm, azopernia, amenorrhoea, alopecia, leucopenia, urinary dysfunction, abdominal cramps, vomiting, diarrhea and severe constipation.
Vindesine (Antiepileptic)	Alopoecia. Granulocytopaenia (dose-limiting); thrombocytopenia, neurotoxicity. Malaise, dizziness, weakness, headache, depression, paraesthesia and numbness, loss of deep tendon reflexes, peripheral neuropathies, constipation, diarrhoea and adynamic ileus; jaw pain and convulsions. Vestibular and auditory toxicity. Rash, nausea and vomiting.
Warfarin (Anticoagulant)	Haemorrhage from almost any organ of the body with consequent effects of haematomas as well as anaemia, tissue necrosis and/or gangrene of skin or other tissues with SC infarction.
Xamoterol (Cardiac stimulant)	Hypotension, bronchospasm, dizziness, headache, palpitation, rashes and muscle cramps.
Xipamide (Antidiuretic)	GI disturbances, hypokalaemia, hyperuricaemia, nocturia, dizziness and impaired glucose metabolism.
Zalcibin (Antiviral)	Hepatic failure; lactic acidosis; pancreatitis; severe hepatomegaly with steatosis
Zidovudine (Antiviral)	Lactic acidosis, severe hepatomegaly with steatosis, hepatotoxicity. Blood dyscrasias, e.g. serious anaemia (may require transfusion), neutropenia and leucopenia.
Zimelidine (Antidepressant)	Hepatic disorders and hypersensitivity reaction.

TABLE 3.2 Contd...

Name of Drugs	Adverse Drug Reactions (ADR)
Zolpidem (Anxiolytic)	Atypical thinking and behaviour, hallucination, nightmare, somnolence, somnambulism, headache, nausea, vomiting, dizziness, vertigo, drowsiness, asthenia, ataxia, rebound insomnia, amnesia, GI disturbances, upper and lower respiratory tract infection, fatigue, visual disturbances, increased ALT serum concentrations and abnormal LFT.
Zopiclone (Hypnotic)	Metallic or bitter after taste; irritability, confusion, depressed mood, aggressiveness, incoordination, anterograde amnesia, mild increase in LFTs, drowsiness, lightheadedness, nausea, vomiting, urticaria and rashes.
Zuclopenthixol (Antipsychotic)	Drowsiness, blurred vision, tachycardia, nausea, dizziness, headache, excitement, postural hypotension, hyperprolactinaemia, sexual dysfunction, ECG changes (prolongation of QT interval and T wave changes), hyperthermia. Extrapyramidal symptoms may occur, especially during the early phase of treatment; urinary frequency or incontinence and tardive dyskinesia.

CHAPTER 4

Good Pharmacovigilance Practice (GPP)

Pharmacovigilance is the science of collecting, monitoring, researching, assessing and evaluating information from healthcare providers and patients on the adverse effects of medications, biological products, herbalism and traditional medicines with a view of identifying new information about hazards associated with medicines and preventing harm to patients[1]. It is basically concerned with the adverse drug reactions. Again, according to World Health Organization (WHO), Pharmacovigilance has been defined as: The science and activities relating to the detection, assessment, understanding and prevention of adverse effects or any other drug related problem.

A pharmaceutical product is launched in the market after being tested and studied through various stages of clinical trials. But such clinical trials have certain number of limitations like patients are selected based upon inclusion-exclusion criteria, limited duration of trials etc. Moreover the clinical trials are conducted under controlled condition and high supervision. The information about the drug that are obtained during the stages of clinical trials or in the premarketing step may not reflect the way it will behave while being used for large populations in hospitals or in general practice. After approval when a variety of patients start taking the medicine new undetected adverse drug reactions, drug interactions, chronic toxicity may come out. In order to find out such undetected threats of the approved drug various post authorization safety studies (PASS) are carried out. These are called post-marketing surveillance.

Pharmacovigilance mainly involve:

- Improve patient care and safety in relation to the use of medicines and all medical and paramedical interventions.
- Enhance public health programmes by collecting good information on the effects of medicines and develop early warning of problems which might affect the success of the programme.

- Discover newer adverse drug reaction while post-marketing surveillance
- Improve public health and safety in relation to the use of medicines.
- Monitoring and collecting data related to Adverse drug reactions
- Analysis of the collected data
- Evaluation of the data
- Organizing public awareness camp to make people aware about adverse drug reactions
- Monitoring data to detect signal
- Detect problems related to the use of medicines and communicate the findings in a timely manner.
- Contribute to the assessment of benefit, harm, effectiveness and risk of medicines, leading to the prevention of harm and maximization of benefit.
- Encourage the safe, rational and more effective (including cost-effective) use of medicines.
- Promote understanding, education and Clinical training in Pharmacovigilance and its effective communication to the public.

Pharmacovigilance involve different kind of people directly or indirectly like

- Patients who use medicines
- Health care professionals like doctors, pharmacists, nurses
- Companies responsible for distribution of medicines
- Pharmaceutical companies or others who work as sponsor
- Regulatory Authorities

Health officials, planners, the staff of pharmacovigilance centres, public health teams and all health workers should become familiar with some factors related with pharmacovigilance, which are-

- *Safety of medicine:* A guide to detecting and reporting adverse drug reactions.
- *The importance of pharmacovigilance:* Safety monitoring of medicinal products.

- *Safety monitoring of medicinal products:* Guidelines for setting up and running a Pharmacovigilance centre.
- *The safety of medicines in public health programmes:* Pharmaco-vigilance is an essential tool.

Terms Related to Pharmacovigilance

Before going into details, various terms related to Pharmacovigilance should be known. Some of them are given below

Adverse event: An **adverse event (AE)** is any untoward medical occurrence in a patient or clinical investigation subject administered a pharmaceutical product and which does not necessarily have a causal relationship with this treatment. An adverse event (AE) can therefore be any unfavorable and unintended sign (including an abnormal laboratory finding), symptom, or disease temporarily associated with the use of a medicinal (investigational) product, whether or not related to the medicinal (investigational) product[2].

Adverse drug reaction: A response to a drug which is noxious and unintended, and which occurs at doses normally used in man for the prophylaxis, diagnosis, or therapy of disease or for the modification of physiological function[3].

Frequency Categories for Adverse Reactions

Very common: > 1/10 • Common: > 1/100 to < 1/10 • Uncommon: > 1/1000 to < 1/100 • Rare: > 1/10000 to < 1/1000 • Very rare: < 1/10000

Clinical trials: Clinical trials are a group of systemic studies with pharmaceutical products or medical device or treatment or preventive measures on human participants to identify pharmacokinetics and pharmacodynamics of the products with the aim of establishing their safety and efficacy. The design of a clinical trial will depend on the drug and the phase of its development. OR

Any investigation in human subjects intended to discover or verify the clinical, pharmacological and/or other pharmacodynamic effects of one or more investigational medicinal product(s), and/or to identify any adverse reactions to one or more investigational medicinal product(s) and/or to study absorption, distribution, metabolism and excretion of one or more investigational medicinal product(s) with the objective of ascertaining its (their) safety and/or efficacy. This includes clinical trials carried out in either one site or multiple sites.

Absolute risk: Risk in a population of exposed persons; the probability of an event affecting members of a particular population (e.g. 1 in 1,000). Absolute risk can be measured over time (*incidence*) or at a given time (prevalence)[4].

Benefit: An estimated gain for an individual or a population[4].

Benefit-risk analysis: Examination of the favorable (beneficial) and unfavorable results of undertaking a specific course of action. (While this phrase is still commonly used, the more logical pairings of benefit-harm and effectiveness-risk are slowly replacing it)[4].

Regulatory authority: The legal authority in any country with the responsibility of regulating all matters relating to drugs[4].

Signal: Reported information on a possible causal relationship between an adverse event and a drug, the relationship being unknown or incompletely documented previously. Usually more than a single report is required to generate a signal, depending upon the seriousness of the event and the quality of the information. The publication of a signal usually implies the need for some kind of review or action[4].

There are three categories of signals: **Confirmed signals** where the data indicate that there is a causal relationship between the drug and the adverse event; **Refuted (or false) signals** where after investigation the data indicate that no causal relationship exists; and **Unconfirmed signals** which require further investigation (more data) such as the conducting of a post-marketing trial to study the issue.

Pharmacovigilance Risk Assessment Committee (PRAC): A Committee of the European Medicines Agency. This committee assess and monitors the safety issues for human medicines[5].

Individual Case Safety Report (ICSR): Information for the reporting of one or several suspected adverse reactions to a medicine that occur in an individual patient at a particular point of time[4].

Marketing Authorization Holder: MAH is an organization who is permitted for marketing the medicinal products for specified indication. It has an appropriate system of Pharmacovigilance in place in order to assure responsibility and liability for its products on the market and to ensure that appropriate action can be taken, when necessary[6].

Periodic Safety Update Report (PSUR): A systematic review of the global safety data which became available to the manufacturer of a marketed drug during a specific time period. Produced in an internationally agreed format[4].

Causality Assessment: One of the most important, and challenging, problems in pharmacovigilance is that of the determination of causality. Causality refers to the relationship of a given adverse event to a specific drug. The evaluation of the likelihood that a medicine was the causative agent of an observed adverse reaction. Causality assessment is usually made according established algorithms[4].

MedDRA: MedDRA is the Medical Dictionary for Regulatory Activities[4]. This dictionary is developed by ICH (International Conference of Harmonization) and it can code for various symptoms like headache, dizziness, asthenia, ischemic attack, influenza, Fanconi-syndrome and many others.

Council for International Organizations of Medical Sciences (CIOMS): It is an international, non-profit, non-government organization sets up working groups to facilitate discussions on policy matters between pharmaceutical industry and drug-regulatory authorities in the field of drug safety. It was found by WHO (World Health Organization) and UNESCO (United Nations Educational, Scientific and Cultural Organization). CIOMS has run a program focusing on drug safety since the early 1980s which incorporates distinct working groups[7].

CIOMS FORM-I*

Among the various guidelines published by CIOMS, CIOMS-I was developed several years ago. This provides a complete format to report adverse drug reaction by any medicinal products.

Spontaneous Reporting: System whereby case reports of adverse drug events are voluntarily submitted from health professionals and pharmaceutical manufacturers to the national regulatory authority.[4] Spontaneous reporting system relies on vigilant physicians and other healthcare professionals who not only generate a suspicion of an ADR, but also report it.

Good Pharmacovigilance Practice: Good Pharmacovigilance practice is the minimum standard for monitoring the safety of medicines on sale to the public in the EU (European Union). The new Pharmacovigilance legislation was introduced by EMEA (European Medicines Evaluation

Agency) in 2012. After the introduction of Good Pharmacovigilance practice the definition of adverse reaction has changed.

CIOMS FORM

| SUSPECT ADVERSE REACTION REPORT | | | |

I. REACTION INFORMATION

1. PATIENT INITIALS (first, last)	1a. COUNTRY	2. DATE OF BIRTH			2a. AGE Years	3. SEX	4-6 REACTION ONSET			8-12 CHECK ALL APPROPRIATE TO ADVERSE REACTION
		Day	Month	Year			Day	Month	Year	

7 + 13 DESCRIBE REACTION(S) (including relevant tests/lab data)

☐ PATIENT DIED

☐ INVOLVED OR PROLONGED INPATIENT HOSPITALISATION

☐ INVOLVED PERSISTENCE OR SIGNIFICANT DISABILITY OR INCAPACITY

☐ LIFE THREATENING

II. SUSPECT DRUG(S) INFORMATION

14. SUSPECT DRUG(S) (include generic name)

20 DID REACTION ABATE AFTER STOPPING DRUG? ☐ YES ☐ NO ☐ NA

15. DAILY DOSE(S)

16. ROUTE(S) OF ADMINISTRATION

21. DID REACTION REAPPEAR AFTER REINTRO-DUCTION? ☐ YES ☐ NO ☐ NA

17. INDICATION(S) FOR USE

18. THERAPY DATES (from/to)

19. THERAPY DURATION

III. CONCOMITANT DRUG(S) AND HISTORY

22. CONCOMITANT DRUG(S) AND DATES OF ADMINISTRATION (exclude those used to treat reaction)

23. OTHER RELEVANT HISTORY (e.g. diagnostics, allergics, pregnancy with last month of period, etc.)

IV. MANUFACTURER INFORMATION

24a. NAME AND ADDRESS OF MANUFACTURER		
	24b. MFR CONTROL NO.	
24c. DATE RECEIVED BY MANUFACTURER	24d. REPORT SOURCE ☐ STUDY ☐ LITERATURE ☐ HEALTH PROFESSIONAL	
DATE OF THIS REPORT	25a. REPORT TYPE ☐ INITIAL ☐ FOLLOWUP	

*Source-http://cioms.ch/index.php/cioms-form-i/Suspect Adverse Reaction Report Form

History & Current Status of Pharmacovigilance

According to different literatures of ancient times, humans were aware of various possibilities of harmful effects of drugs and other medical procedures. Different medical schools were also empowered to inspect adulteration. The oath of Apothecaries was first to mention a statement about the use of drugs by physician in 13th century. In 18th century people became more aware about safety issues related to drugs as physicians came to know numerous more severe adverse drug reactions. Both the physicians and academicians started publishing papers and giving lectures on topics related to safe use of drugs. The "thalidomide disaster" occurred in 1961 when nearly 12000 children were found to have congenital abnormalities due to maternal use of thalidomide.[8,9] The thalidomide incident was so tragic that several systemic approaches were made for routine monitoring and collecting reports related to adverse drug reaction. Deaths of many people due to altered composition of digitalis tablet (0.25 mg of digoxin instead of 0.05 mg) in 1971 also made an alarming notice[10]. In 1971, during 20th World health assembly an International Drug Monitoring Program occurred and the current Pharmacovigilance system of the national Pharmacovigilance centres were established in 1972. The centre works by collaborating with WHO. The requirement for developing the importance of Pharmacovigilance had led to the establishment of Council for International Organizations of Medical Sciences. This organization provides various guidelines relating to Pharmacovigilance. International Conference on Harmonization was also established. World Health Organization along with all other organizations work together for improvising the system of Pharmacovigilance.

The concept of developing Pharmacovigilance centres was first proposed in 1986 in India. Pharmacovigilance centres were first established in pharmacology department of All India Institute of Medical Sciences (AIIMS). Failure of this program due to various reasons had led to establishment of a new National Pharmacovigilance Program sponsored by WHO and funded by World bank. Central Drugs Standard Control Organizations (CDSCO) is also a part of NPP. There are two zonal centres (South-west zonal Centre in Department of Clinical Pharmacology, Seth GS Medical Collage and KEM Hospital, Mumbai and North-east zonal Centre in the Department of Pharmacology, AIIMS, New Delhi), five regional centres and twenty four peripheral centers under this program which collect information about Adverse drug reaction. The information gathered by these centres is sent to the NPAC and to the UMC in Sweden.

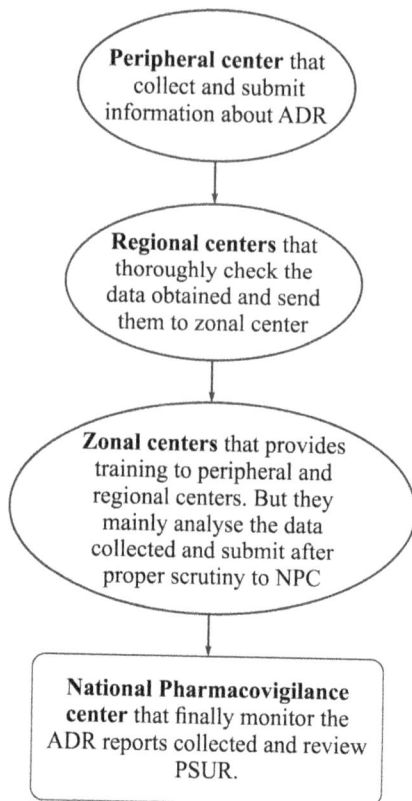

Fig. 4.1 Work Flow of Different Pharmacovigilance centres.

The Pharmacovigilance System

Monitoring of safety profile of medicines and detection of any change in their risk-benefit profile are carried out by establishing a Pharmacovigilance system. The Pharmacovigilance system allows other organizations to carry out legal responsibilities related to Pharmacovigilance.

The old system: Before July 2012, there was an old regulation that had been followed in Pharmacovigilance system. In old system, according to European Union, each Marketing Authorization Application (MAA) had to include a detailed description of the Pharmacovigilance System, including a named EU Qualified Person for Pharmacovigilance. The details of the style of the old system were documented within Volume 9a of "the rules governing medicinal products in the European Union." The responsibilities, roles and activities related to Pharmacovigilance are well described in it.

The new system: The new Pharmacovigilance legislation has become effective from July 02, 2012. The concept of good Pharmacovigilance practices has provided a well-defined framework within which the new Pharmacovigilance system works. The underlying objectives of the applicable EU legislation for Pharmacovigilance are:

- Preventing harm from adverse reactions in humans arising from the use of authorized medicinal products within or outside the terms of marketing authorization or from occupational exposure[11].

- Promoting the safe and effective use of medicinal products, in particular through providing timely information about the safety of medicinal products to patients, healthcare professionals and the public. Pharmacovigilance is therefore an activity contributing to the protection of patients' and public health[11].

Good vigilance practice has made certain changes in different area. In the old system reporting was not centralized as reports had to be submitted to each regulatory authority. After introduction of Good Pharmacovigilance practice only EMEA-Eudravigilance was liable to collect all reports. The definition of adverse reaction also changed.

A response to a medicinal product which is noxious and unintended.

Before Good Pharmacovigilance practice: Which occurs at doses normally used in man. After Good Pharmacovigilance practice:-which occurs within or outside the marketing authorization condition or from occupational exposure.

The responsibilities of Marketing authorization holder, the format of PSUR also changed.

Pharmacovigilance system master file: The pharmacovigilance system master file is a legal requirement that was first introduced by the European Union to successfully manage the requirements to conduct several pharmacovigilance activities. The process and content of pharmacovigilance system master file is applicable irrespective of the structure of marketing authorization holder, the residence of the qualified person responsible for pharmacovigilance. It must be available within the European Union. This master file contains all details related to training, planning of inspections and audit, planning of risk management, safety profiles, signal management, regulatory framework, the detail qualification and responsibilities of the qualified person for pharmacovigilance etc. Due to establishment of pharmacovigilance system master file, the marketing authorization holders (MAH) and the qualified person has become able to find the compliance and non-compliance of the system, the flaws and deficiencies of pharmacovigilance system, to confirm that the system has been implemented according to the requirements. The pharmacovigilance system master file should have different sections like section on qualified person responsible for pharmacovigilance (QPPV) describing the responsibilities of the person to promote satisfied pharmacovigilance system along with the Curriculum vitae, contact details and also the backup system to be followed in absence of the authorized qualified person. It should have section on sources on safety data, computerized system and databases (Eudravigilance), quality system, pharmacovigilance processes, pharmacovigilance system processes[12]. The pharmacovigilance system master file is located within the European Union and is available both in electronic format and paper-based format.

Eudravigilance: Eudravigilance is a data processing network and management system for reporting and evaluating suspected adverse drug reactions (ADRs) during the development, and following the marketing authorization of medicinal products in the European Economic Area (EEA). The first operating version was launched in December 2001.

Eudravigilance supports:

- The electronic exchange of suspected adverse drug reaction reports known as Individual Case Safety Reports) between the European Medicines Agency (EMA), National Competent Authorities (NCAs), Marketing Authorization Holders (MAHs), and sponsors of clinical trials in the EEA.

- Early detection of possible safety signals associated with medicinal products for human use.

- Continual monitoring and evaluation of potential safety issues in relation to reported adverse reactions.

- Decision making process, based on a broader knowledge of the adverse reaction profile of medicinal products especially in the form of Risk Management.

Taking into account the pharmacovigilance activities in the pre- and post- authorization phase, Eudravigilance provides two reporting modules:

- *The Eudravigilance Clinical Trial Module (EVCTM)* to facilitate the electronic reporting of Suspected Unexpected Serious Adverse Reactions (SUSARs) as required by Directive 2001/20/EC and
- *The Eudravigilance Post-Authorization Module (EVPM)* for post-authorization Individual Case Safety Reports (ICSRs) as required by Regulation (EC) No 726/2004, Directive 2001/83/EC as amended.[13]

Qualified Person for Pharmacovigilance (QPPV): There is a qualified person in the European Union who should have knowledge about every aspect of pharmacovigilance. Marketing authorization holders mainly need this person. This person is involved with the preparation and maintenance of reports of adverse drug reactions, periodic safety update reports and other reports related to pharmacovigilance.

Background and Development of Good Pharmacovigilance Practice[11,14]

To facilitate the performance and to put more importance on Pharmacovigilance system new legislation was introduced by the European Union in July 2012. Good Pharmacovigilance practice is new set of guidelines that provide framework for smooth running of Pharmacovigilance. It has replaced the old style of Pharmacovigilance system in volume 9A of "The rules governing medicinal products in the European Union". Good Pharmacovigilance practice is divided into two sectors

- Modules of Pharmacovigilance Practices
- Product or population specific consideration

Modules of Good Pharmacovigilance Practice:

Module I	Pharmacovigilance Systems and their quality systems
Module II	Pharmacovigilance system master file (PSMF)
Module III	Pharmacovigilance inspections
Module IV	Pharmacovigilance audits
Module V	Risk management systems
Module VI	Management and reporting of adverse reactions

Contd...

Module VII	Periodic safety update report
Module VIII	Post-authorization safety studies
Module VIII Addendum I	Member States' requirements for transmission of information on non-interventional post authorization safety studies
Module IX	Signal Management
Module X	Additional Monitoring
Module XI	Public participation in Pharmacovigilance
Module XII	Continuous pharmacovigilance, ongoing benefit-risk evaluation, regulatory action and planning of public communication
Module XIV	International cooperation
Module XV	Safety communication
Module XVI	Risk-minimization measures: selection of tools and effectiveness indicators
Module XVI Addendum I	Educational materials

* The module numbers XI, XII, XIII and XIV stay void, as their planned topics have been addressed by other guidance documents on the Agency's website.

Final Good Pharmacovigilance Practice Annex:

Annex-I	Definitions
Annex-II	Templates
Annex-III	Other Pharmacovigilance guidelines
Annex-IV	International Conference on Harmonization of Technical Requirements for Registration of Pharmaceuticals for Human Use (ICH) guidelines for pharmacovigilance
Annex V	Abbreviations

GVP product- or population-specific considerations:

| Product- or population-specific considerations I | Vaccines for prophylaxis against infectious diseases |

The modules of pharmacovigilance processes are developed by a team consisting of expert members from EMEA and EU. All modules of good vigilance practices did not develop at the same time. The first seven modules were taken into consultation between February to April 2012 and after considering the comment from stakeholders it was finally available from July 02, 2012. Module III and Module IV were finally published in December 2012. Good pharmacovigilance practice annex-I was also published with it. The final module XV and good pharmacovigilance practice annex-II also published together in January

2013.The final module X was published in April 2013. Some modules have been revised as final like module II was published in its first revision in April, 2013. On June 2013 the draft revision I of module VI was released for consultation. Another draft revision of module XVI was published in June 2013. Both the modules were published finally in 2014. Revision I of module V and revision I of module III was published in 2014 in April and September consecutively. The first chapter with product or population specific considerations was provided in its first revision on December, 2013.

Only the stakeholders and members of European Union can make any correction, addition or deletion to the content of guidelines of good pharmacovigilance practices. Other organizations and people related to pharmacovigilance can only send proposal of changes to authorized website of European Union. European Union has an expert team who goes through the proposals and takes necessary actions whether to implement the changes or not. Each chapter of good pharmacovigilance practice has two sections. Section A provides the legal and technical issues while section B focus on guidelines.

Conclusion

The world has seen several terrific incidents due to use of drugs in human being. Pharmacovigilance is the only fruitful system which can reduce the risk of disasters due to use of drugs. It is good that a system has been developed including all types of health care professionals to allow them work properly for pharmacovigilance. Good pharmacovigilance practice is a novel procedure to make pharmacovigilance system more valid and successful worldwide, but the gap between the established policy and work procedure maintaining the proper policy need to be filled to establish an effective pharmacovigilance system. More countries need to be involved in this program to make it effective.

References

1. CIOMS. (undated). Drug Development and Use. [online] CIOMS. Available at:http://www.cioms.ch/about/frame_drug_development.html

2. Guideline on good pharmacovigilance practices (GVP): Module II – Pharmacovigilance system master file (Rev 1). European Medicines Agency. 9 April 2013,EMA/816573/2011 Rev 1*

3. Guidelines on good pharmacovigilance practices (GVP): Introductory cover note, last updated with launch of public consultation of addendum I to module XVI on educational materials. European Medicines Agency. 27 April 2015,EMA/239760/2015

4. http://eudravigilance.ema.europa.eu/human/index.asp

5. http://www.ema.europa.eu/ema/index.jsp?curl=pages/about_us/general/gen eral_content_000537.jsp

6. ICH GCP

7. Lely AH. Digital is intoxicate, waarnemingenbetreffendeeenmassale digitoxine-intoxicate teVeenendaal. Thesis. State University of Groningen. Stafleu. Leiden, 1971.

8. Randell T. Thalidomide's back in the news, but in more favorable circumstances. JAMA,1990; 263:467-68.

9. Source.http://www.ema.europa.eu/ema/index.jsp?curl=pages/regulation/doc ument_listing/document_listing_000345.jsp

10. Source-The European Agency for the evaluation of medicinal products, 1999.

11. Surada Prakash Rao, "Importance of Pharmacovigilance in Indian Pharmaceutical Industry"Asian Journal of Research in Pharmaceutical Sciences 10/2011; 2(1):4-8.

12. Wade OL. The dawn of concern. In: Adverse reactions to drugs: 1-10. Acford Ltd. Chichester,1970

13. WHO 1972

14. who-umc.org/Graphics/24729/glossery of terms used in pharmacovigilance.

CHAPTER 5

Pharmacovigilance- An update of Global and Indian Scenario

Pharmacovigilance is defined as the science and activities relating to detection, assessment, understanding and prevention of adverse effects or any other drug related problem. At the end of 2010, 134 countries were part of WHO pharmacovigilance programme. The aim of pharmacovigilance is to enhance patient care and patient safety in relation to the use of medicines, and to support public health programme, by providing reliable, balanced information for the effective assessment of the risk benefit profile of medicines.

The WHO programme for international drug monitoring provides a forum for WHO member states to collaborate in pharmacovigilance. WHO, Geneva, is responsible for policy issues while the operational responsibility rests with Uppsala Monitoring Centre (UMC) Sweden.

Considering the sensitive nature of the data being collected within the programme, countries contributing such data to the scheme have agreed on certain requirements that should be complied by countries wishing to join collaboration with WHO, being an organization for co-operation between member states requires administrative structure in pharmacovigilance activity. The basic requirements are

(i) General acquaintance with the methodology of spontaneous monitoring

(ii) A national centre for Drug Monitoring must be designated and recognized by Ministry of health

(iii) Technical Competence to fulfill reporting requirements to WHO

(iv) Practical procedure for joining the WHO drug monitoring programme

The practice of monitoring the effects of medical drugs after they have been licensed for use, specially in order to identify and evaluate previously unreported adverse reaction.

It is also known as drug safety in the Pharmacological Science relating to the collection, detection, assessment, monitoring and prevention of adverse effects products.

Aims and Scopes

1. To improve the patient care and safety in relation to medical and paramedical intervention.
2. To improve the public health and safety in relation to the use of medicines for public health.
3. To contribute to the assessment of benefit, harm, effectiveness and risk of medicines
4. To promote understanding, clinical training and effective communication to health professionals and public community.

Pharmacovigilance, as outsourcing industry existed for ten years in India and has evolved from functional outsourcing of case processing to full service providers of pharmacovigilance activities for an entire molecule or therapeutic area.

Standardization of safety data: Drug safety focus has been shifted to comply the ever increasing regulatory guideline in developed markets. Efficient resource management is commonly achieved by specific roles that are present with the organization. Drug safety is collaborating with other functions like clinical, regulatory affairs and quality assurance. Standardization of safety data by utilization of E2B guidelines of ICH has been proved successful. This E2B is applicable to other functions like clinical, regulatory affairs and quality assurance for processing the incoming and outgoing data. Data on adverse events (AE) is collected within organizations and outside like social media. The safety data is to ensure regulatory compliance and clarity about the meaning for patient safety and product quality. If an organization has a number of products under development, there is a need to focus on risk management.

The pharmacovigilance input into product development is guided by development safety update report (DSUR) and Risk Management Plan (RMP). Pharmacovigilance is a part of product development programme and the clinician should be aware of the ratio of risk and benefit for the product. The documented aspect of risk-benefit ratio should be addressed throughout the development programme. This will help for the preparation of risk management plan and reduce the queries related to post authorization safety and efficacy studies. Post marketing authorization involves the reports of risk management plans. Post authorization safety studies is a requirement for approval in marketing authorization (MA).

Cross functional expertise is the best option for relevant expertise from pharmaceutical, clinical and pharmacovigilance. The overall responsibilities include protocol development, study management, documentation etc.

Pharmacovigilance system master file- This is documentation related to continuous monitoring of risk- benefit profile.

Inter- Relationship between Pharmacovigilance and Public Health Programme

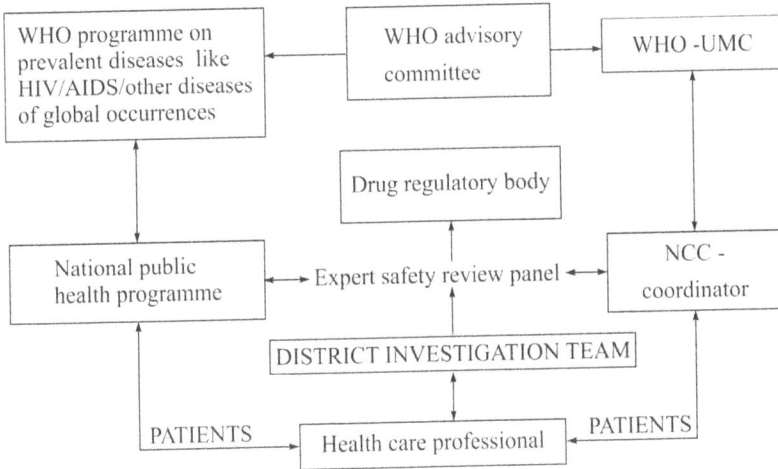

Fig. 5.1 Integrated approach of pharmacovigilance with public health programme[1].

The sustainability of public health programme depends on good pharmacovigilance. In many countries, public health departments functions at different levels as primary, district, state or country level.

The use of pharmaceutical preparation is one of the fastest growing components of healthcare budget. At the same time, adverse reactions are significant cause of morbidity and mortality. The treatment of adverse drug reactions (ADR) imposes financial burden due to medical intervention and hospitalization. Healthcare professionals share their experience to enrich the understanding about underlying principles of disease and medicines.

Requirements for Pharmacovigilance in Public Health Programme (PHP)

The principal objectives of pharmacovigilance in public health:

(a) Rational and safe use of medicines by healthcare professionals.

(b) Assessment and communication of the risks and effectiveness of medicine used

(c) Educating and informing patients

Pharmacovigilance system must be capable for following important functions:

(a) Receiving and processing of reports

(b) Establishing databases, data analysis and review

(c) Decision making, risk management and follow up

(d) Communication and co-ordination between pharmacovigilance, regulatory and public health activities

(e) Training in all aspects of pharmacovigilance

(f) International linkage

The pharmacovigilance in public health team must address above functionalities and submit clear organograms specifying roles and responsibilities (National state District Primary health centre Village) will vary between countries and depend on existing healthcare and regulatory norms of the country.

Data Collection, Investigation and Management of Adverse Reaction

The following people and organizations are important:

(a) Patient

(b) Primary healthcare professionals

(c) District hospital and Healthcare officer

(d) Investigation team

(e) Tertiary care- referral hospitals

(f) Programme managers

(g) National pharmacovigilance coordinator

(h) Expert safety review panel

The village health worker or physician at primary health centre, along with district health officer, programme manager and the tertiary care referral hospital constitute the team for detection, investigation, tackling and reporting ADR's.

It is needless to mention that ADR's be reported as soon as possible.

Minor suspected ADR's should be tackled by primary healthcare workers. Serious areas should be taken to the newest hospitals for the investigation and management. People from Public Health Programme (PHP) are best suited for detection, investigation and management of ADR's.

Co-ordination

Co-ordination and integration of pharmacovigilance activity between different disease specific public health programme.

The co-ordinator should be member of expert safety review panel and selected from pharmacovigilance centre. This person should be knowledgeable about pharmacovigilance and able to develop a national pharmacovigilance system as per international standard.

Expert Safety Review Panel

The panel is comprised of

(a) Programme manager

(b) Pharmacovigilance co-ordinator

(c) Clinical Pharmacologist

(d) Pharmaceutical Scientist

(e) Members from specialized discipline like Gynecologist etc

Functions of the Panel

(i) Review reports sent by Programme Manager

(ii) Evaluate safety issues from ADR reports

(iii) Evaluate reports originated from lack of efficacy

(iv) Recommend further investigation

(v) Recommend appropriate actions

The data base: The data base is necessary for reported case assessment, analysis and follow up. The data base includes:

(a) Site of report generation
(b) Identity of the reporter
(c) Identity of the patient
(d) Demographic details of the patient
(e) Information about the concerned medicine, name and the formulation, manufacturer, mode of administration, dose and dates of administration.
(f) All relevant information about structured product labeling norms (SPL)
(g) Concomitant medication with dose, dates and indication.
(h) Assessment of seriousness
(i) Management and outcome

In case of special situation like pregnancy, the national pharmacovigilance coordinator has to maintain registrar and report all observation to expert panel.

Similarly, all deaths related to medicines must be reported to expert panel.

Decision making: Medicine regulatory authority with the inputs from expert panel, national pharmacovigilance center, national public health programme, WHO collaborating center for international Drug Monitoring, WHO and International advisory panel provides the necessary advice.

International linkage and data base: Whenever a pharmacovigilance center is organized in a country, it should be linked to WHO international network of pharmacovigilance centers. Experience from public health programmes will fortify WHO database.

Spontaneous reporting: Reports of adverse drug reactions are voluntarily submitted by health care professionals, pharmaceutical companies or the users to the national pharmacovigilance centers.

Responsibilities:

(a) *Patients and the public:* Due to patient awareness about adverse reactions, early reporting and taking appropriate actions are important.

(b) *Primary healthcare professionals:* Primary healthcare staff should detect, investigate, manage and report adverse drug reactions. Following approaches are considered for effective reporting:

   (i) Easy availability of reporting forms

   (ii) Acknowledgement of receipt of the report and provision of feedback to the reporter

   (iii) Participation of reporting staff in professional meetings

   (iv) Collaboration with national pharmacovigilance center

(c) *District investigation team:* This team should

   (i) Review all reports

   (ii) Screen the reports for further investigation on the basis of seriousness including death, severity, exposure to medicine during pregnancy

(d) *National pharmacovigilance co-ordinator:* Responsibilities include coordination, communication, integration, training and supervision of pharmacovigilance activities of district investigation team. This person is responsible for collection and storage of all reports of adverse reactions and co-ordination between national pharmacovigilance center, the district investigation team, the public health programme at national level, the ministry of health, international centers and pharmaceutical manufacturer. The coordinator should process ADR reports for assessment by expert safety review panel.

ADR reports are categorized as

   (i) Reports screened by district investigation team for further consideration

   (ii) Reports concerning about a signal of new adverse reaction

   (iii) Overall profile of the medicines can be studied

Pharmaceutical Industry

They are responsible for the quality and safety of medicines when they are available in market. They have also a duty to assess the safety and effectiveness on public health programme and the benefits of the patient.

The national public health and pharmacovigilance programme: National Pharmacovigilance Center, in association with public health programme decides the priorities and establish the linkage with WHO for technical and policy matters.

The media: The media contribute effectively through the awareness development in the community. Media can open a channel with experts to ensure the authentic information required to dispel any misconception about medicines and thereby the problem can be tackled effectively to regain public confidence.

The role of WHO and international advisory committee: WHO acts as a repository of information from pharmacovigilance programme and public health programme. WHO responds to all queries, debates and controversies regarding the safety of medicines.

WHO provides the leadership in training and capacity development.

The advisory committee promotes the future development of pharmacovigilance as an important subject.

Training and Capacity Building

Public health professionals lack the knowledge and expertise to deal with the drug induced disease, unexpected adverse reactions, adverse reactions to new drugs and adverse reactions to the vulnerable sections of patients like pregnant women, paediatric and geriatric groups.

Evaluation of the System

Assessment of Pharmacovigilance System

The criteria are as follows:

(i) Distribution of the reporting of the professionals or patient reporting

(ii) Complete and precise information

(iii) Promptness of reporting

(iv) Rate of reporting

(v) Impact of adverse reactions in terms of hospital admission due to adverse drug reactions.

Apart for the above evaluation parameters, there is a need to conduct studies for the evaluation of impact on pharmacovigilance in public health

Good Pharmacovigilance Practice

Successful pharmacovigilance relies on contribution from people with varying educational background. Since the health professionals, patients and public at large are unaware of pharmacovigilance. Standard operating Procedures (SOP) should provide information.

(i)   What is a reportable adverse reaction?

(ii) What is to report a suspected medicine related problem?

(iii) The availability of filling a reporting form

(iv) Procedure for collection of reports

(v)   Routines for assessment processing of case report at the pharmacovigilance centre

(vi) Procedures for analysis and aggregated information and option for action

(vii) Good communication practices

(viii) Monitoring system should be provided by performance indication.

As the development of medicine is going on rapid pace, WHO promotes the use of new medicines to control diseases along with industry participation. The approach of ADR monitoring is changing for this reason.

Strength and Weakness of Pharmacovigilance and Public Health Programme

Strength: Strength of Pharmacovigilance programme lies in the development of new methods for the assessment of safety of medicines. The Pharmacovigilance programme assess quality, efficacy of the medicine including the correct indications for use.

Another strength in Pharmacovigilance programme is the training and expertise in benefit-risk evaluation and its communication to the people at large.

The early identification and prevention of adverse reactions leads to more rational use of medicines within target patient group. The procurement of medicines can be based on above rational judgement.

Finally, resources and information base can be shared so that duplication of effort can be avoided.

Weakness: Insufficient resources are inadequate for training and capacity building. Inadequate funding is also deterrent for drug efficacy and safety monitoring.

Detection and management of ADR are perceived to have negative meaning on public health programmes. The information from public health programme is not always added to international database for Pharmacovigilance. As a result, the regulators do not have the benefit of feedback concerning medicines used in public health programmes.

Scenario of Public Health Environment in India

Lack of good evidence and training programmes for health care professional in developing countries like India, patients are at a risk of medication error and adverse drug reaction.

The risk factors are:

1. Disease
2. Population
3. Medicines (counterfeit, substandard, donated, medicine interactions, incorrect use of medicines)
4. Healthcare Provider
5. Healthcare System

Disease: In developing countries like India, treatments started in absence of elaborate diagnosis and insufficient follow-up of patients.

Population: Public health programmes provide services to large population. Treatment could be extended to patients who are predisposed towards contra-indication. These groups of patients are known as vulnerable group.

Medicines: In developing countries like India, Government agencies are not in a position to exert proper grip on medicines with doubtful quality. In rural and semi-urban areas, access to medicinal product is not always through professional healthcare people, but through pharmacies and pseudo- professional people.

Counterfeit medicines: Widespread use of medicine which are not genuine including life saving drugs like antibiotics is the cause of treatment failure and fatalities at times. Patients taking counterfeit medicines unknowingly do not get intended benefits and face complicated situations. In one reported case, the placebo tablets were sold as contraceptive medicine leading to unwanted pregnancy.

Substandard medicines: In case of generic drugs and their formulations, it has been found occasionally that certain percentage of medicines do not comply with quality control tests and specifications. The non compliance can be attributed to non-GMP manufacturing method, improper packaging and storage. Sometimes, failure can occur in dissolution testing, and uniformity of dosage parameter also.

Death cases have been reported in case of diethylene glycol contamination in liquid oral formulation[5]. This product is an accompanying impurity with Poly ethylene glycol which is an important solvent for many drugs in liquid oral formulation, particularly for paediatric use. So polyethylene glycols must be tested before use for the content of diethylene glycol.

Donated medicines: These medicines were found to be either not complying with the quality standards or it is expired. Such medicines are bound to cause adverse drug reactions. WHO guidelines suggest

(a) Maximum benefit to user

(b) Respect and good will for recipient

(c) No double standard on quality

(d) Effective communication between donor and recipient

Performance Indicators Related to Pharmacovigilance

The detection of signal and their evaluation, the safety database outputs, interactions with clinical departments reveal

1. Risk management system and tracking of risk minimization measures. These activities are of cross functional nature and all such interactions must be well documented.

2. Periodic safety update reporting (PSUR) scheduling, production and submission

3. Communication of safety concerns to consumers, healthcare professionals and competent authorities.

4. Implementation of safety information to summary of product characteristics (SPC) and patient information leaflet.

Specific key performance indicator for individual areas related to pharmacovigilance as well as the holistic network and infrastructure of the system. This includes the general awareness amongst all the members of the organization about reporting safety information and those involved in safety information are trained and competent enough to make the right decision for the patient and society at large.

In 2010, Pharmacovigilance programme of India (PVPI) has been set up for monitoring adverse drug reactions (ADR) and assure the benefits of drugs takes prevalence over risks.

Indian Pharmacopoeia Commission (IPC) started functioning as national co-ordination center (NCC) for PVPI since 2011.

Signal detection is an important vertical of Pharmacovigilance. Signal review panel under the PVPI has been formed by ministry of health and family welfare to study the relationship between adverse effect and a drug with available database. (causality assessment). Since PVPI is the source of available database for Indian drug regulators, continuous training programmes and research are undertaken by NCC-PVPI.

There is a need to have a detailed pharmacovigilance study report for the drugs of longer use like anti-tubercular, anti- retrovirals, anti diabetic, anti hypertensive etc. Information on the incidence, time of onset, clinical symptoms to observe as predictive of serious harmful signals, stopping, restarting, risk factors, dose calculations as seen in Indian population needs to be compiled and used for formatting guidelines.

The PVPI reports need to be compiled. The signals of new ADRs due to variation in prescribing practices, risk factors should be recorded.

The National Pharmacovigilance Programme will have the following Milestone:

1. *Short- term objectives:* To foster a culture of notification
2. *Medium-term objectives:* To engage several healthcare professional and Non Government Organizations (NGOs) in drug monitoring and information dissemination process.
3. *Long-term Objectives:* To achieve such professional efficiencies that would make Indian Pharmacovigilance programme a benchmark for drug monitoring endeavours.
4. *Periodic safety update reports:* These shall be expected to be submitted every 6 months for the first two years of marketing in India, and annually for the subsequent 2 years. In addition, training programmes and interaction meetings to be held every 6 months after the initial training.

The Pharmacovigilance effort in India is coordinated by The Pharmacopoeia Commission and conducted by the Central drugs Standard Control Organization (CDSCO).

The main responsibility of the IPC is to maintain and develop the Pharmacovigilance data base consisting of all suspected serious to medicines observed.

Indian Pharmacopoeia Commission (IPC) is functioning as National Coordination Center (NCC) for Pharmacovigilance Programme of India (PVPI). NCC is operating under the supervision of steering committee which recommends procedures and guidelines for regulatory interventions. The main responsibility of NCC is to monitor all the adverse reactions of medicines being observed in the Indian Population and to develop and maintain its own Pharmacovigilance database.

The aim of the commission that acts like the National Coordination Center (NCC) for PVPI is for the safety of the patient, safety of the population with respect to the user of the Drug.

The Government of India have made a separate, dedicated, autonomous institution in the form the Indian Pharmacopoeia commission (IPC) to deal with matters relating to timely publication of the Indian Pharmacopoeia which is the official book of standards for drugs and formulations specifying the standards of identity, purity and strength of the drugs imported, manufactured for sale, stocked or exhibited for sale or distribution in India.

The commission is supposed to perform functions such as revision and publication of the Indian Pharmacopoeia and National formulary of India, providing IP reference standards and training to the stakeholders on pharmacopoeial issues. The commission has become operational from January 2009 as an autonomous body under the administrative control of Ministry of Health and Family Welfare.

The Central Drugs Standards Control Organization (CDSCO), in collaboration with IPC, Ghaziabad is initiating a nation-wide Pharmacovigilance Programme for protecting the health of the patients by assuring drug safety. The programme shall be coordinated by IPC, Ghaziabad as a National Coordinating Centre (NCC). The centre will operate under the supervision of the steering committee.

Background

The PVPI was initiated by Government of India in July 2010 with the All India Institute of Medical sciences (AIIMS), New Delhi as the NCC for monitoring Adverse Drug Reactions (ADRs) in the country for protecting Public Health. In the year 2010, 22 ADR monitoring centers including AIIMs, New Delhi was set up under this programme. The NCC was shifted from AIIMS New Delhi to IPC, Ghaziabad in April 2011.

Scope

Before registration and marketing of medicines in the country, its safety and efficacy is evaluated in clinical trials. These trials mainly detect common adverse reactions. Some adverse reactions which takes a long time to develop, may not be detected in clinical trials. Besides, the control conditions maintained in clinical trials do not reflect the usage pattern in practice. For a medicine considered to be safe, its expected benefits should be greater than associated risks of harmful reactions. So, a continuous post marketing monitoring system or pharmacovigilance is essential to know a comprehensive safety profile of medicine. These include spontaneous ADR reporting, action taken by regulatory authorities in other countries.

Since adverse drug reactions carry social and economic consideration, there is a need to employ healthcare professional (HCP) and the public at large for monitoring adverse drug reactions in the country.

Committee under PVPI

The programme is administered and monitored by Steering committee. Collection of ADR reports are to be made from MCI approved medical colleges and hospitals, Private hospitals, Public health programmes and Autonomous Institutions like ICMR etc.

Mission: To safeguard the health of the Indian population by monitoring the drug safety and reducing the risk associated with its use.

Vision: To improve the patient safety and welfare in Indian population by monitoring the drug safety and risk associated with the medicines.

Objectives:

- To create a nation-wide system for patient safety reporting
- To identify and analyse the new signal (ADR) from the reported cases
- To analyse the benefit- risk ratio of marketed medicines
- To generate evidence based information on safety of medicines
- To support regulatory agencies in the decision- making process on the use of medications

- To communicate the safety information on the use of medicines to various stake holders to minimise the risk
- To emerge as a National center of excellence for pharmacovigilance activities
- To collaborate with other national centers for the exchange of information and data management
- To provide training and consultancy support to the national pharmacovigilance center located across the globe

Implementation of PvPI

In India with a population of over 1.25 billion with a vast ethnic variability, difference disease prevalence pattern, practice of different systems of medicines, different socioeconomic strata, it was important to have a standardized and powerful pharmacovigilance and drug safety monitoring programme for the nation.

Collaboration with WHO – Uppsala Monitoring Centre (UMC)

WHO and UMC work with 130+ countries worldwide. The long term objective of the PvPI is to establish a centre of excellence for Pharmacovigilance in India. In this direction, the PvPI-NCC will collaborate with the WHO-UMC based in Sweden. The responsibilities of WHO-UMC towards NCC are as follows:

1. Training of the staff at the PvPI-NCC at IPC-Ghaziabad, the ADRs Monitoring centres in medical colleges across the country.
2. Usage of UMC developed Vigiflow software for medicines at no cost to PvPI
3. Access to Vigibase, which contains worldwide medicines safety data.
4. Access to early information about potential safety hazards of medicines.
5. Technical collaboration for PvPI
6. Technical collaboration for a regular publication that will be issued by the PvPI-NCC for the distribution to the ADR monitoring centers and other stakeholders.
7. CDSCO headquarters are in continuous liaison with UMC for the technical collaboration.

WHO- UMC & INDIA

The WHO programme for International Drug Monitoring provides a forum for WHO member states that includes India to collaborate in the monitoring of drug safety. Within the program, individual case reports of suspected adverse drug reactions are collected and stored in a common database, presently over 3.7 million case reports.

Since 1978, the Uppsala Monitoring centre (UMC) in Sweden has carried out the program. The Uppsala Monitoring Centre is responsible for the collection of data about adverse drug reactions around the world, especially from countries which are the members of the WHO including India. Member countries send their reports to the UMC where they are being processed, evaluated and entered into the WHO international database. There are several reports of adverse reactions to a particular drug. A signal is being detected which reflects the possibility of a hazard that is further communicated to member countries. This happens only after detailed evaluation and expert review. Through membership of The WHO international Drug monitoring programme, a country can come to know if similar reports are being made elsewhere. Despite the fact that India is a country with large patient population and healthcare professionals, ADR reporting is yet to develop as per international standard.

Table 5.1 Responsibilities of the stakeholders in the programme

Functions of the Stakeholders	
ADRs Monitoring Centre	• Collection of ADR reports • Perform follow up with the complainant to check completeness as per SOPs. • Data entry into Vigi- flow • Reporting to PvPI-NCC through Vigi-flow with the original data along with each ADR case. • Training/sensitization/ feedback to physicians by PvPI-NCC.
PvPI-ADR Monitoring centre like pharmaceutical Industry, corporate hospitals, autonomous institutes	• Collection of ADR reports • Perform follow-up with the complainant • Completeness as per SOP • Report the data to CDSCO-Headquarter
PvPI-NCC, IPC-Ghaziabad	• Preparation of SOPs, guidance documents & training manuals • Data compilation, Relationship assessment as per SOPs.

TABLE 5.1 *Contd...*

Functions of the Stakeholders	
	• Conduct training workshops for all centres. • Publication of medicine safety newsletters. • Reporting to CDSCO-HQ • Analysis of post marketing surveillance, periodic update safety report received from CDSCO-HQ
CDSCO-HQ, NewDelhi	• Appropriate regulatory decision making & actions on the recommendation of PvPI-NCC at IPC-Ghaziabad • Collaboration with WHO-UMC at Sweden • Dissemination of medicine safety related decisions to stakeholders. • Provide for budgetary provisions & administrative support to run PvPI

Roles & Responsibilities of PvPI Personnel at ADR Monitoring Centre

1. At PvPI-AMC,the centre coordinator is responsible for the proper functioning of AMC.

2. The technical associate appointed by NCC will be responsible for the collection and follow up of ADRs, which is to be AMC co-ordinator. All scrutinized and signed reports should be entered in Vigi-flow. Every report has to be sent to NCC for evaluation.

3. Collection, relationship (causality) assessment and scrutinizing the ADR report received will be done as per SOPs by co-ordinator.

4. The centre coordinator is responsible for sending the monthly reports of their AMC to NCC.

5. The Centre coordinator should take initiative to motivate doctors/healthcare professionals/students/ patients of the hospitals for ADR reporting.

6. Feedback to all HCPs engaged in reporting should be sent by centre coordinator.

Roles & Responsibilities of PvPI Personnel at NCC

1. The NCC personnel will be responsible for reviewing ADR reports, to perform quality checks, relationship assessment and ADR reports sent by AMC to WHO-UMC.

2. Monitoring ADR reports entered in Vigi-Flow by AMCs and day to day reports will be sent to AMCs on weekly basis.

3. Cumulative centrewise status report will be sent to AMCs on monthly basis.

4. Generation of reports at periodic intervals required by signal review panel and steering committee.

5. Signal detection and reporting to signal review committee.

6. Review the drugs for focused monitoring (ADR) suggested by CDSCO

7. Publication of safety newsletter on bi-annual basis.

8. Reporting to CDSCO about the functional status of AMCs.

Roles & Responsibilities of PvPI Personnel at Zonal CDSCO Offices

1. Zonal offices provide administrative support to ADR monitoring centres.

2. Distribution of funds for office expenditures incurred by AMCs.

Roles & Responsibilities of PvPI personnel at CDSCO-HQ

1. The annual budget and expansion plan for PVPI are worked out by CDSCO.

2. The decision of the steering committee on NCC reports will be forwarded to CDSCO

3. The CDSCO will report to Drug Technical Advisory Board under Ministry of Health & Family Welfare.

4. The CDSCO is responsible to formulate and communicate safety related regulatory decisions for medicines.

List of CDSCO Zonal and Sub- Zonal Offices

1	CDSCO Zone (Ahmedabad)		
2	CDSCO Zone (Hyderabad)		
3	CDSCO North Zone (Ghaziabad)	1	Sub-zone Office, Chandigarh
		2	Sub Zone Office, Jammu
		3	IGI airport Office, Delhi
4	CDSCO East Zone,(Kolkata)	4	Sea &Airport office, Kolkata

Contd...

5	CDSCO west Zone (Mumbai)	5	Sea & Airport office, Mumbai
		6	JNPT Port Office, Navi Mumbai
6	CDSCO South Zone (Chennai)	7	Sea & Airport Office, Chennai
		8	Sub-Zone & Port Office, Bangalore
		9	Kochi Port Office

Periodic Safety Update Report (PSUR)

The PSUR for marketed drugs was designed to be a stand alone document which allows a periodic but comprehensive assessment global safety data of a marketed drug or biological product. The steps are involved in the PSUR process include adverse drug reaction information, case processing, data retrieval and analysis, medical review and risk assessment. PSUR can be important source for identifying new safety signals, means of monitoring changes in the benefit- risk profile. It is an indicator of the need for risk management initiatives.

In India, PSURs submitted by pharmaceutical companies shall be expected to be submitted every six months for the first two years of marketing in India and annually for subsequent two years. ICH guidelines (E2C) are available on Clinical safety Data management and PSURs for Marketed Drugs.

The proposed contents of PSURs are as follows:

1. Introduction
2. Worldwide market authorization
3. Update on regulatory authority regarding the actions taken for safety reasons.
4. Changes in the reference safety information
5. Patient Exposure
6. Presentation of individual case histories
7. Overall safety evaluation
8. Conclusion

The PSUR process comprises the following steps:

1. Intake of Adverse Drug Reactions (ADR) information.
2. Case Processing
3. Data Retrieval

4. Data Analysis

5. Medical review and risk assessment

In general, safety issues should be identified at an early stage and incorporated in risk management plan. This plan proposes different corrective actions through adopting education of all concerned, systematic marketing approach and utilization of safety database.

Data mining: A computational method to collate the relevant information from a large data pool. In principle, the WHO collaborating centre for International Drug Monitoring has been doing data mining since 30 years using an early relational database. Data mining is considered as a powerful tool in pharmacovigilance.

The Representation of Pharmacovigilance Systems

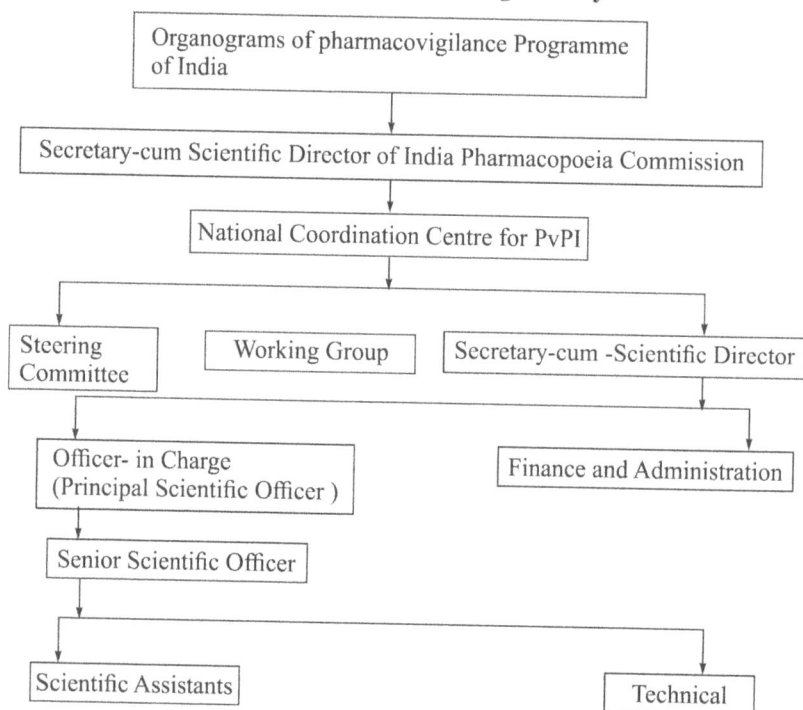

Organograms of pharmacovigilance Programme of India

Secretary-cum Scientific Director of India Pharmacopoeia Commission

National Coordination Centre for PvPI

Steering Committee	Working Group	Secretary-cum -Scientific Director

Officer- in Charge (Principal Scientific Officer)	Finance and Administration

Senior Scientific Officer

Scientific Assistants	Technical

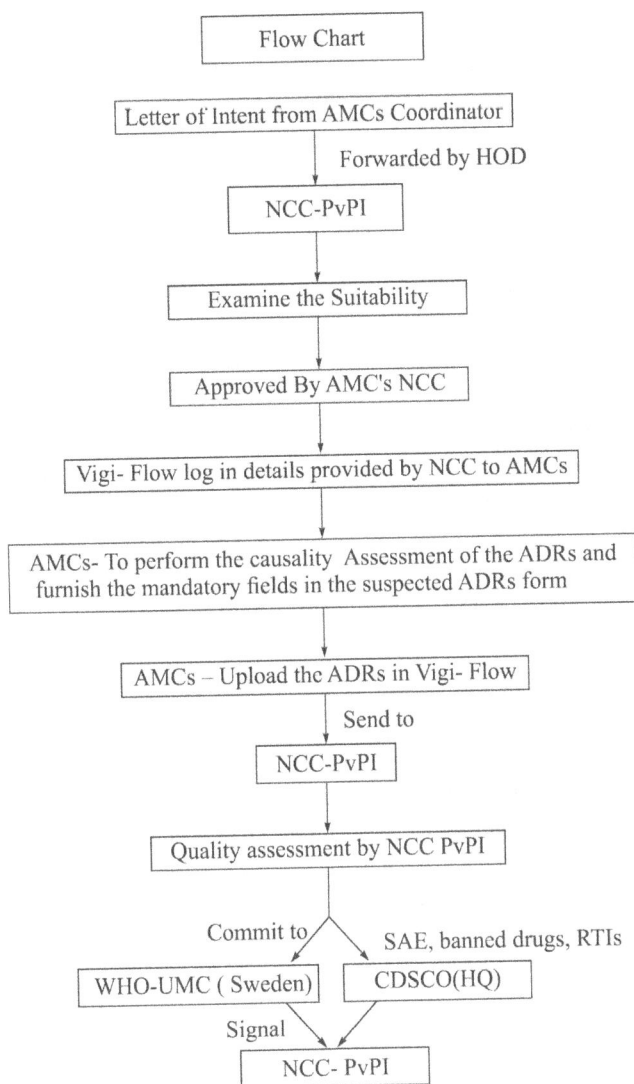

Flow Chart

Letter of Intent from AMCs Coordinator

Forwarded by HOD

NCC-PvPI

Examine the Suitability

Approved By AMC's NCC

Vigi- Flow log in details provided by NCC to AMCs

AMCs- To perform the causality Assessment of the ADRs and furnish the mandatory fields in the suspected ADRs form

AMCs – Upload the ADRs in Vigi- Flow

Send to

NCC-PvPI

Quality assessment by NCC PvPI

Commit to   SAE, banned drugs, RTIs

WHO-UMC (Sweden)	CDSCO(HQ)

Signal

NCC- PvPI

References

1. Aheme GW, Briggs R: The relevance of the presence of certain steroids in the aquatic environment. J. Pharm. Pharmacol 1989, 41: 735-736.

2. Almenoff J, Tonning JM, Gould AL, et al Perspectives on the use of data mining in pharmacovigilance. Drug Saf. 2005, 28: 981-1007.

3. Benichou Ch. ed. Adverse drug reactions- a practical guide to diagnosis and management. Chichester, Wiley & Sons, 1994.

4. Brahmachari B, Fernandes M, Bhatt A Pharmacovigilance for clinical trials in India.: current practice and areas for reform. Perspect clin Res. 2011: 2(2): 49-53.

5. Council for International Organisations of Medical Sciences Benefit - risk balance for marketed drugs: evaluating safety signals. Report of CIOMS Working Group IV. GENEVA, CIOMS, 1998.No.762.

6. Counterfeit Medicines: guidelines for the development of measures to combat counterfeit medicines. Geneva, World Health Organization, 1999 (WHO/EDM/QSM/99.1).

7. Daughton CG, Ruhoy IS. The afterlife of drugs and the role of Pharma-Ecovigilance. Drug saf. 2008: 31(12): 1069-82.

8. David. J. Graham, syed Ahmad and Tony Piazza-HEPP Office of Drug Safety, Center for Drug Evaluation and Research, US Food and Drug Administration, Rockville, MD,USA.

9. Dialogue in Pharmacovigilance- more effective communication. Uppsala, Sweden, Uppsala Monitoring Centre, 2002.

10. Fong, P (2002). Anti depressants in aquatic organisms: a wide range of effects in pharmaceuticals and personal care products in the environment: Scientific and Regulatory issues, eds C. Daugton C.G. and T. Jones-Lapp, 264-281, Washington D.C.: American Chemical Society.

11. ICH Guidelines E2A, E2C, E2D and E6.

12. J.M. Bernardo et al, Bayesian Methods in Pharmacovigilance: Bayesian Statistics, Oxford University Press, 2010.

13. Jonca Bull, Office of the Drug Safety, US Food and Drug Administration, Rockville, MD, USA.

14. Klepper MJ, Integrated Safety Systems Inc, North Carolina, USA.

15. Kshirsagar N, Fermer R, Figueroa BA, GhalibH, LazdinJ. Pharmacovigilance methods in public health programmes; the example of miltefosin and visceral leishmaniasis. Trans R Soc Trop Med Hyg. 2011: 105: 61-7.

16. Kshirsagar N. The Pharmacovigilance system in India. Drug saf. 2005: 28: 647-50.

17. Lazarou J, Pomeranz BH, Corey PN. Incidence of Adverse Drug Reactions in hospitalized patients: a meta-analysis of prospective

studies. Journal of the American Medical association, 1998, 279: 1200-1205.

18. Mann R, Andrews E., eds. Pharmacovigilance, Chichester, Wiley & Sons, 2002.

19. Patrice Verpillat, Department of Special Projects, Lund beck SAS, Paris, France.

20. Pharmacovigilance Programme of India (PvPI)- Published by Indian Pharmacoepia Commission, Ministry of Health and Family Welfare.

21. Pharmacovigilance: A Practical Approach to Reshaping patient Safety, Krishnan Rajagopalan.

22. Richard Williams T, Cook Jon C, Exposure to Pharmaceuticals Present in the Environment. Drug Information Journal 2007, 41(2): 133-141.

23. Safety monitoring of medicinal products- WHO Guidelines for setting up and running a pharmacovigilance center. Stora Torget 3, Uppsala, Sweden, The Uppsala Monitoring Centre, 2000.

24. Sarah Davis, Britget King and June.M.Raine.

25. Singh J, et al. Diethylene glycol poisoning in Gurgaon India 1998 Bulletin of the World Health Organization, 2001,79: 88-95.

26. Sumpter John P. Environmental effects of Human Pharmaceuticals. Drug Information Journal 2007: 41: 143-147.

27. Surveillance of adverse events following immunization (AEFI)- Field guide for managers of immunization programmes (WHO/EPI/ TRAM/93.02 Rev.1).

28. Tandon VR, Mahajan V, Khajuria V, Gillani Z. Under reporting of adverse drug reactions: a challenge for pharmacovigilance in India. Indian J Pharmacol 2015:47 65-71.

29. The safety of medicines in public health programmes: Pharmaco-vigilance an essential tool   WHO 2006.

30. The importance of pharmacovigilance: safety monitoring of medicinal products. Geneva, World Health Organisation, 2002. Vigilance and Risk Management o Medicines, Medicines and healthcare Products Regulatory & Agency, London, UK.

31. WHO Guidelines for Good Donation Practices Revised 1999. WHO/EDM/PAR/99.4. World Health Organization, 1999.

32. Zuccato Ettore, Calamari Davide, Natangelo Marco, Fanelli Roberto: Presence of therapeutic drugs in the environment. The lancet 2000, 355: 1789-1790.

APPENDIX

Table 1 Approved New Drugs in India

The following drugs were approved during the period of
April to June 2016 by CDSCO

Sl No.	Drug	Indication
1	TofacitinibTablets 5 mg	To treat adult patients with Moderately to severely active rheumatoid arthritis who have had an inadequate response or intolerance to Methotrexate. It may be used as monotherapy or in combination with methotrexate or other non-biological Disease modifying antirheumatic drugs (DMARDs)
2	Ceftaroline Fosamil Injection 600 mg/vial	For the treatment of adult (>18 years of age) patients with community-acquired pneumonia.
3	Panobinostat Hard Gelatin Capsules 10 mg/15 mg/20 mg (Panobinostat lactate)	In combination with Bortezomib and dexamethasone, is indicated for the treatment of multiple myeloma, who have received at least 1 prior therapy
4	Bepotastine Besilate Bulk & Bepotastine Besilate 1.5% w/v Ophthalmic solution	For the treatment of itching associated with allergic conjunctivitis
5	Ibutilide Bulk & Amp; Ibutilide Fumarate Injection 0.1 mg/ml	For the rapid conversion of atrial fibrillation or atrial flutter of recent onset to sinus rhythm. Patient with atrial arrhythmias of longer duration are less likely to respond to Ibutilide Fumarate Injection. The effectiveness of Ibutilide has not been determined in patients with arrhythmias of more than 90 days in duration.

Table 2 WHO Scale (ADR)

Term	Description
Certain	A Clinical event, including laboratory test abnormality, occurring in a plausible time relationship to drug administration, and which cannot be explained by concurrent disease or other drugs or chemicals. The response to withdrawal of the drug (dechallenge) should be clinically plausible. The event must be definitive pharmacologically or phenomenologically, using a satisfactory rechallenge procedure if necessary.
Probable/ Likely	A Clinical event, including laboratory test abnormality, with a reasonable time sequence to administration of the drug, unlikely to be attributed to concurrent disease or other drugs or chemicals, and which follows a clinically reasonable response on withdrawal (dechallenge). Rechallange information is not required to fulfill this definition.
Possible	A Clinical event, including laboratory test abnormality, with a reasonable time sequence to administration of the drug,but which could also be explained by concurrent disease or other drugs or chemicals. Information on drug withdrawal may be lacking or unclear.
Unlikely	A Clinical event, including laboratory test abnormality, with a temporal relationship to drug administration which makes a causal relationship improbable, and in which other drugs, chemicals or underlying disease provide plausible explanations.
Conditional/ Unclassified	A Clinical event, including laboratory test abnormality, reported as an adverse reaction, about which more data is essential for a proper assessment or the additional data are under examination.
Unassessable/ Unclassifiable	A report suggesting an adverse reaction which cannot be judged because information is insufficient or contradictory, and which cannot be supplemented or verified.

Table 3 Naranjo Scale (ADR)

TOTAL: (1-4: POSSIBLY; 5-8: PROBABLY; > 9: DEFINITELY)

Questions	Yes	No	Don't know
Were their previous conclusive reports on this reaction?	-1	0	0
Did the adverse event appear after the suspected drug was administered?	+2	-1	0
Did the adverse reaction improve when the drug was discontinued or specific antagonist was administered?	+1	0	0
Did the adverse drug reaction reappear when the drug was readministered?	+2	+1	0
Are their alternative causes (other than the drug) that could have caused the reaction?	-1	+2	0
Did the reaction reappear when a placebo was given?	-1	+1	0
Was the drug detected in the blood (or other body fluids) in a concentration known to be toxic?	+1	0	0
Was the reaction more severe when the dose was increased, or less severe when the dose was decreased?	+1	0	0
Did the patient have a similar reaction to the same or similar drugs in any previous exposure?	+1	0	0
Was the event confirmed by objective evidence?	+1	0	0

Table 4 P$_v$PI Drug Safety Alerts (APRIL-JUNE 2016)

The preliminary analysis of suspected Unexpected Serious Adverse Reactions (SUSARs) from PvPI ICSRs database reveals that following drugs are associated with the risks

ROFLUMILAST
Indication: Reduce the risk of Chronic Obstructive Pulmonary Disease Exacerbation
Alert: Gynaecomastia

CLOZAPINE
Indication: Management of Schizophrenic patients.
Alert: Neutropenia

DISULFIRAM
Indication: Alcohol abuse deterrent
Alert:
Erythroderma

PEGINTERFERON ALPHA
Indication: Chronic active hepatitis B & C
Alert: Vasculitis

PIPERACILLIN & TAZOBACTAM
Indication: In the treatment of lower Respiratory tract infection/Urinary tract infection/intra abdominal infections, Skin and skin structure infections, Bacterial septicaemia involving polymicrobic infection.
Alert: Blurred vision

MOMETASONE FUROATE, TOPICAL
Indication: Steroidal responsive dermatitis, Eczema/Atopic dermatitis
Alert: Hypertrichosis/Hirsutism, Skin Depigmentation

AMPHOTERICIN B (Conventional)
Indication: Life threatening fungal infections including Histoplasmosis, Coccidioidomycosis, Paracoccidioidomycosis, Blastomycosis, Aspergillosis, Cryptococcosis, Mucormycosis, Sporotrichosis and candidiasis; Visceral and mucocutaneous leishmaniasis unresponsive to pentavalent antimony compounds; Severe meningitis, Perioral Candidiasis.
Alert: Bone marrow depression

RANIBIZUMAB
Indication: Neovascular Age-related Macular Degeneration (AMD), Visual impairment due to Diabtic macular Edema (DME), Visual impairment due to Choroidal Neovascularization secondary to Pathologic Myopia (PM)
Alert: Myocardial Infarction

DOXORUBICIN
Indication: Soft tissue and bone Sarcomas, Acute leukemia, Malignant lymphoma, Hodgkin's disease, Breast Carcinoma, Small cell carcinoma of lungs, AIDS-related kaposi's sarcoma, Multiple myeloma, Gastrointestinal tract carcinoma, Bladder cancer, Ovarian carcinoma, Acute myeloblastic leukemia, Thyroid carcinoma, Neuroblastoma.
Alert: Photosensitivity Reaction

CRIZOTINIB
Indication: Locally advanced or Metastatic Non-small cell Lung Cancer (NSCLC) that is Anaplastic Lymphoma kinase (ALK) positive
Alert: Pneumonitis, Hepatic Encephalopathy

Table 5 New AMCS launched in P$_v$PI

State	Centre name	Coordinator Name & Designation
Andhrapradesh	Rangaraya Medical College, Kakinada, AndhraPradesh-533001	Dr. K. V. Siva Prasad (Prof. Pharmacology)
	Konaseema Institute of Medical Sciences and Research Foundation & KIMS General Hospitals, Chaitanya Health City, Amalapuram, East Godavari District- 533201, AndhraPradesh	Dr. Anand Acharya (Prof. & HOD Pharmacology)
Karnataka	Shri B.M Patil Medical College, BLDE University, Vijayapur-586103,Karnataka	Dr. Anant Khot (Asst. Prof. Pharmacology)
	Shivamogga Institute of Medical Sciences, Sagar Road, Shivamogga-577201, Karnataka	Dr. S. Nagaraja Prasad (Asst. Prof. Pharmacology)
	M. R. Medical College, Kalaburagi-585105	Dr. Santosh Kumar Jeevangi (Prof. Pharmacology)
Kerala	Sree Gokulam Medical College & Research Foundation (S. G.M.C & R.F), Venjaramoodu, Thiruvanthapuram, kerala-695607	Dr. P. Shobha (Assoc. Prof. Pharmacology)
Tamilnadu	Kanyakumari Govt. Medical College, Asaripallam, Kanyakumari, District- 629201, TamilNadu	Dr. T Ashok Kumar (Prof. & HOD Pharmacology)
Puducherry	Pondicherry Institute of Medical Sciences, Ganapathichettikulam, kalapet, Pondicherry-605014	Dr. Manjunatha C H (Asst. Prof. Pharmacology)
Bihar	M. G. Memorial Medical College, Purabbali, Dinajpur Road, Kishanganj, Bihar-855107	Dr. Rabindra Nath Chatterjee (Professor- Pharmacology)
Uttarpradesh	Teerthankar Mahaveer Medical College and Research Centre, N.H-24, bagarpur, Delhi Road, Moradabad, UP-244001	Dr. Prithpal Singh Matreja (Prof. & HOD Pharmacology)
	Yashoda Super Speciality Hospital, H-1, Kaushambi, Ghaziabad-201010	Dr. G.J Singh (Sr. Consultant, Medicine)
	National Drug Dependence Treatment Centre (NDDTC), Sector-19, KamalaNehru Nagar, C. G.O Complex,Ghaziabad-201002	Dr. Sudhir K Khandelwal (Prof. & HOD, Centre Chief)

TABLE 5 *Contd...*

State	Centre name	Coordinator Name & Designation
Chattisgarh	C.M. Medical College and Hospital, Vill & P.O: Kachandur, Durg, Chattisgarh-490024	Dr. Sunita Chanrekar (Prof. & HOD Pharmacology)
Delhi	Institute of Liver and Biliary sciences (ILBS), D-1, Vasant Kunj, New Delhi-110070	Dr. Davesh Gupta (Assistant Professor, Clinical Research)
Westbengal	ICARE Institute of Medical Sciences & Research and Dr. Bidhan Chandra Roy Hospital, Banbishnupur, Balughata, Haldia, dist- Purba Medinipur, WB-721645	Dr. Sukanta Sen (Assoc. Prof., Pharmacology)
Maharashtra	Jawaharlal Nehru Medical College, Datta Meghe Institute of Medical Sciences, Sawangi (Meghe), wardha-442004	Dr. Sailesh Nagpura (Asst. Professor)
	Aswini Rural Medical College, Hospital & Research Centre, Kumbhari, Tq South Solapur-413006	Dr. C.S. Waghmare (Prof. & HOD Pharmacology)
	Terna Medical College & Hospital, Sector-12, Phase-II, Nerul, Navi Mumbai-400706, Maharashtra	Dr. Sangita Sukumaran (Prof. & HOD Pharmacology)
	SMedical Smt. Kashibai Navale Medical College & General Hospital, Sr. No. 49/1, narhe, Off Mumbai-Pune bypass, Pune-411401	Dr. Yogita karandikar (Assoc. Prof., Pharmacology)
Madhyapradesh	Gajra Raja Medical College, Veer Savarkar Marg, Gwalior, M.P- 474009	Dr. Saroj Kothari (Prof. & HOD Pharmacology)
Gujrat	Smt. Bhikhiben Kanjibhai shah (SKBS), Medical Institute & Research Centre, At. & P.O, Piparia, Tal. Waghodia, Dist. Vadodara- 391760	Dr. B.M Sattigiri (Prof. & HOD Pharmacology)
Rajasthan	Dr. S N Medical College, Residency Road, Shastri Nagar, Jodhpur-342001	Dr. Anusuya Gehlot (Senior Prof. Pharmacology)

Table 6 Suspected Adverse Drug Reaction Reporting Form

For VOLUNTARY reporting of Adverse Drug Reactions by healthcare professionals

CDSCO **Central Drugs Standard Control Organization** Directorate General of Health Services, Ministry of Health & Family Welfare, Government of India, FDA Bhavan, ITO, Kotla Road, New Delhi www.cdsco.nic.in	AMC/ NCC Use only AMC Report No. Worldwide Unique no.

A. Patient Information	12. Relevant tests / laboratory data with dates
1. Patient Initials	2. Age at time of Event or date of birth / 3. Sex ☐ M ☐ F / 4. Weight ___ Kgs	

B. Suspected Adverse Reaction

5. Date of reaction stated (dd/mm/yyyy)

6. Date of recovery (dd/mm/yyyy)

7. Describe reaction or problem

13. Other relevant history including pre-existing medical conditions (e.g. allergies, race, pregnancy, smoking, alcohol use, hepatic/ renal dysfunction etc)

14. Seriousness of the reaction

Death (dd/mm/yyyy) ___   Congenital anomaly
Life threatening   Required intervention
Hospitalization-initial or   to prevent permanent
    prolonged   impairment / damage
Disability   Other (specify)

15. Outcomes

Fatal   Recovering   Unknown
Continuing   Recovered   Other (specify)

C. Suspected medication(s)

S No	8. Name (brand and /or generic name)	Manufactu rer (if known)	Batch No / Lot no (if known)	Exp. Date (if known)	Dose used	Route used	Frequency	Therapy dates (if known give duration) Date started	Date stopped	Reason for use of prescribed for
i.										
ii.										
iii.										
iv.										

Sl No As per C	9. Reaction abated after drug stopped or dose reduced					10. Reaction reappeared after reintroduction				
	Yes	No	Unknown	NA	Reduced dose	Yes	No	Unknown	NA	If reintroduced dose
i.										
ii.										
iii.										
iv.										

11. Concomitant medical product including self medication and herbal remedies with therapy dates (exclude those used to treat reaction)	D. Reporter (see confidentiality section in first page) 16. Name and Professional Address : Pin code : E-mail Tel. No. (with STD code) Occupation Signature 17. Causality Assessment 18. Date of this report (dd/mm/yyyy)

www.ingramcontent.com/pod-product-compliance
Lightning Source LLC
Chambersburg PA
CBHW050656190326
41458CB00008B/2588